20th Century Jewelry

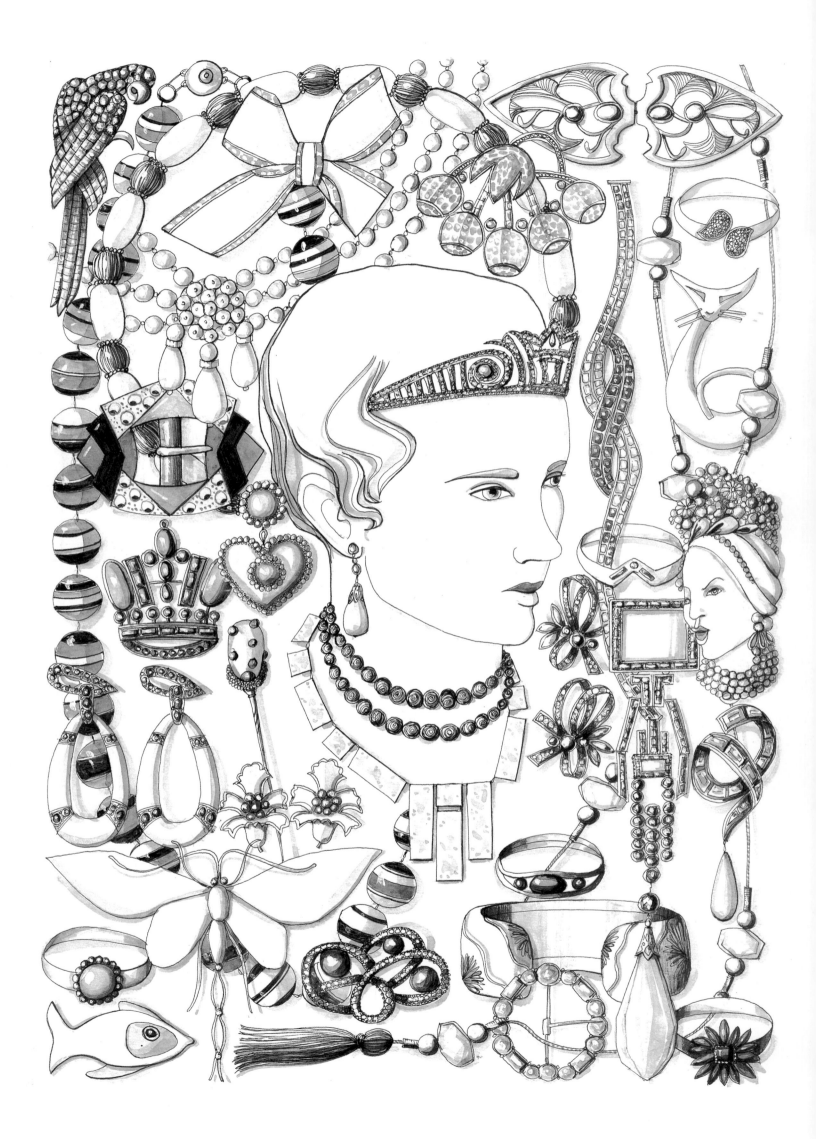

John Peacock

20th Century Jewelry

The Complete Sourcebook

with over 1,500 color illustrations

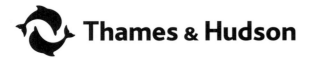

Thames & Hudson

To Hanna Worrall

© 2002 Thames & Hudson Ltd, London

First published in hardcover in the United States of America
in 2002 by Thames & Hudson Inc., 500 Fifth Avenue,
New York, New York 10110

thamesandhudsonusa.com

Library of Congress Catalog Card Number 2001099704
ISBN 0-500-51083-0

Printed and bound in China by Midas Printing

Contents

Introduction

In *20th Century Jewelry* my aim has been to illustrate as many types and styles of jewelry as possible, both real and imitation, concentrating on those which I consider to be of most interest and usefulness to the designer, student, enthusiast and non-specialist to whom this book is directed. The term 'jewelry' includes here any decorative article, made from any material, which is intended to be worn as personal adornment, whether hung, pinned or clipped on to the body (such as a necklace, bangle or earring) or pinned, clipped or sewn on to clothing (such as a brooch, pin or beaded motif). Also included are jewelled and beaded garments, as well as functional objects such as buckles, hatpins, haircombs, tiepins and cufflinks. Ornamental watchcases, pendant and lapel watches, and wristwatches are also shown.

The styles presented are, in the main, those worn by fashionable women and men of their time, though I have on occasion chosen to illustrate interesting or unusual pieces in the style of famous twentieth-century designers, where I feel these to be informative and appropriate. To set the jewelry in its context, I have on most pages included a figure presenting the overall fashionable look of each period.

The collection is divided into five parts of sixteen pages each. Each section covers a twenty-year duration and each decade is allotted seven pages, grouped under headings such as 'Brooches', 'Earrings', 'Necklaces', 'Bracelets', 'Rings', 'Buckles and Clasps' and 'Hair Ornaments'. Because some pieces of jewelry appear less consistently than others, these headings vary somewhat for each period. Necklaces, for example, remain constant throughout, but in the 1950s their popularity was such that more than one page was needed to illustrate the range of styles. Other pieces come and go: hair ornaments, for instance – an essential accessory for the lady of the 1900s – dwindled into obscurity by the 1930s, only to come to life again in the 1950s. Similarly, novelty jewelry was relatively rare in the early years of the century, but became more dominant among the cocktail jewelry of the 1940s. And in the latter decades of the century such a wide variety of earrings was worn that extra space has had to be allocated to them in the book.

The main titles are followed by a page covering two decades, headed 'Miscellaneous Jewelry and Jewelled Pieces'. This encompasses watches, jewelled belts, scarf rings, garniture and the like. Jewelry items worn by men were fewer and their changes were less radical: these are therefore confined to a single page at the end of each twenty-year period. Each section is followed by eight pages of schematic drawings and detailed descriptions of each piece of jewelry.

The division between real jewelry and fashion or costume jewelry has never been a clear one. Take, for example, snail shells bound with gold wire to form a brooch or earrings, or tortoiseshell inlaid with gold forming a pendant suspended from a gold chain. Both these pieces include an element of precious metal, but the remaining components would not be deemed precious or real. In the drawings I have not differentiated between real, precious, fake, costume or fashion jewelry but have made clear in the explanatory notes which objects contain real gems and which include fake, imitation, glass or plastic stones. I have also distinguished between those that are made from gold or other precious metals and those that are not.

At the beginning of the century fine jewelry designers adopted a new, elegant style known as Belle Epoque, inspired by the eighteenth century, which featured fine pierced trelliswork and loops, swags and garlands of stylized flowers with diamonds and pearls set in platinum. Art Nouveau designers, also at the turn of the century, took ideas directly from nature and executed them in materials chosen for their aesthetic rather than intrinsic value, such as ivory, tortoiseshell and horn. After the First World War the Art Deco style came into fashion. Art Deco owed nothing to tradition and little to nature but was closely associated with contemporary art, the machine age and the streamlined architecture of the time. A revival of Egyptian-style jewelry also took place in the 1920s, following the discovery early in the decade of Tutankhamun's tomb: large and elaborate gold pieces with multicoloured patterns became popular, as did designs incorporating scarab beetles and lotus flowers.

The 1930s saw the evolution of more feminine jewelry, with figurative, foliate and floral influences. Marcasite was fashionable, often teamed with jade, coral, cornelian or chrysoprase. During this decade, and continuing into the 1940s, novelty jewelry was much in demand, made either from precious components or from materials such as plastic, stamped or pressed base metal or wood. These pieces often took the form of animals and birds, stylized flowers and fruit, or fruit-laden Carmen Miranda heads and dancing figures. At the end of the 1930s cocktail jewelry began to take centre stage and it became even more prevalent in the 1940s. This was robust, assertive jewelry, with ribbon-like loops and voluptuous curves and fan shapes in bright yellow gold set with cascades of real or fake rubies, sapphires, aquamarines and amethysts.

Towards the end of the 1940s and throughout the 1950s witty figurative motifs and cartoon-style animals were the vogue, along with fruit, flowers and vegetables (particularly mushrooms), scarecrows and ballet dancers. All could be found with precious stones set in platinum or gold, or with faceted glass stones set in gold-coloured base metal. During the latter part of the 1950s a trend towards free and relaxed 'modern' jewelry prevailed – asymmetric slabs of gold offset with brightly coloured cabochon stones, or semi-precious stones in their polished but uncut form. In this period more self-consciously 'modern' jewelry also began to be produced and continued in popularity into the 1960s, when natural, organic shapes and molten-looking metal were set with uncut crystals or semi-precious stones such as tiger's eye, lapis lazuli or onyx.

In the 1960s designers also began to look to the past for inspiration; some were drawn to expensive, larger-than-life pieces. For young 'swingers' there was Op Art jewelry, often in stark black and white or with brightly coloured geometric patterns. Bangles and earrings were frequently made from luminous transparent or opaque plastic. The 1970s witnessed a fashion for more minimal jewelry, with fine outlines set with small stones, or strong shapes coloured with enamels, though hippies favoured ethnic and handmade pieces. At the end of the decade there was also a fashion for large flower brooches and for rigid bangles and necklaces.

In the early 1980s outsized Maltese-style crosses set with multicoloured stones made their appearance, hand-in-hand with a revival of out-and-out glamour, sometimes referred to as 'Retro Chic'. Glittery, sparkling and showy, this jewelry was worn at any time of day, breaking all the rules of previous decades which stated that 'a lady should never wear diamonds in daylight'. By the mid-1990s classical retrospective styles were back, this time with a more subtle approach, and by 1999 there was a rich and varied range of real, imitation, fake, fashion and costume jewelry in both period and modern styles.

At the end of this book a chart of the development of twentieth-century jewelry outlines at a glance the principal changes that took place throughout the period in some of jewelry's main items: earrings, brooches, rings, necklaces and pendants, and bracelets and bangles. These changes were often brought about by jewelry designers and companies who pushed jewelry design forward by introducing new styles, shapes and materials. Such innovators include not only fine jewellers, like Cartier, Tiffany and Bulgari, but also costume jewellers like Trifari and Miriam Haskell, and what are sometimes known as 'art jewellers', like René Lalique and Line Vautrin. Brief biographies and histories of some of these designers and companies appear at the end of this book. In addition, a bibliography lists those works which have been especially useful in compiling this survey.

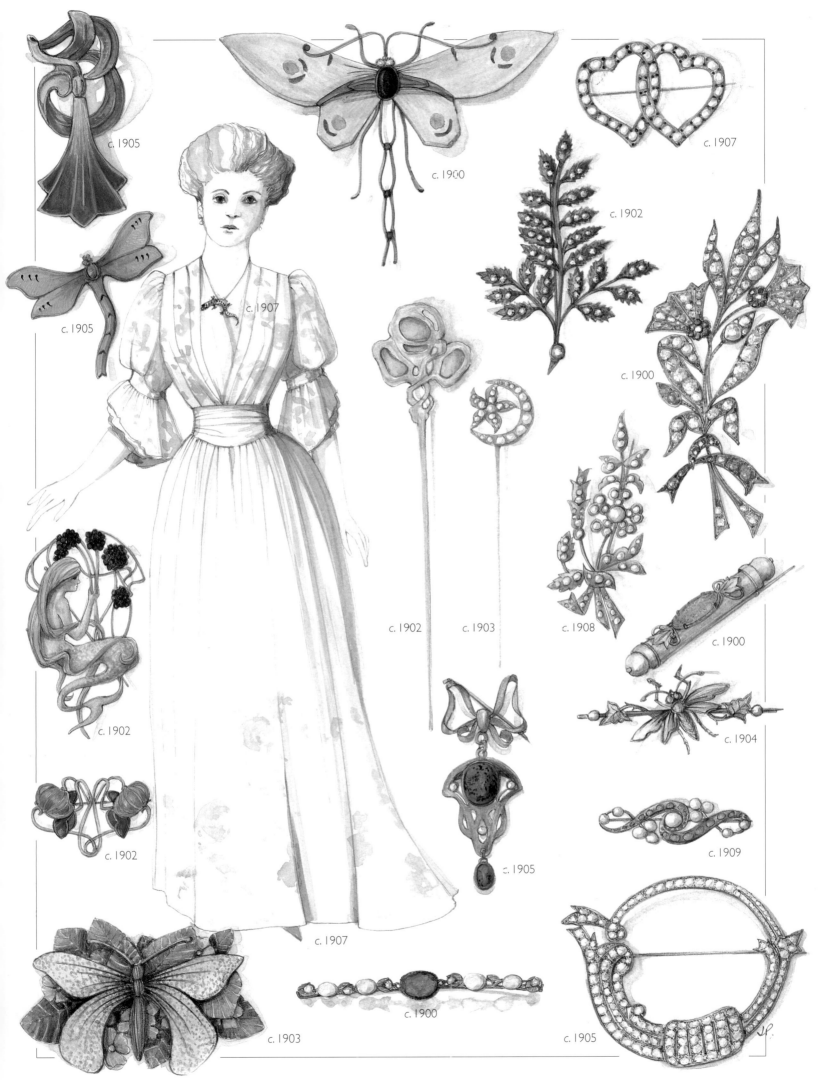

c. 1905

c. 1900

c. 1907

c. 1902

c. 1905

c. 1907

c. 1900

c. 1902

c. 1902

c. 1903

c. 1908

c. 1900

c. 1904

c. 1902

c. 1905

c. 1909

c. 1907

c. 1903

c. 1900

c. 1905

Earrings 1900–1909

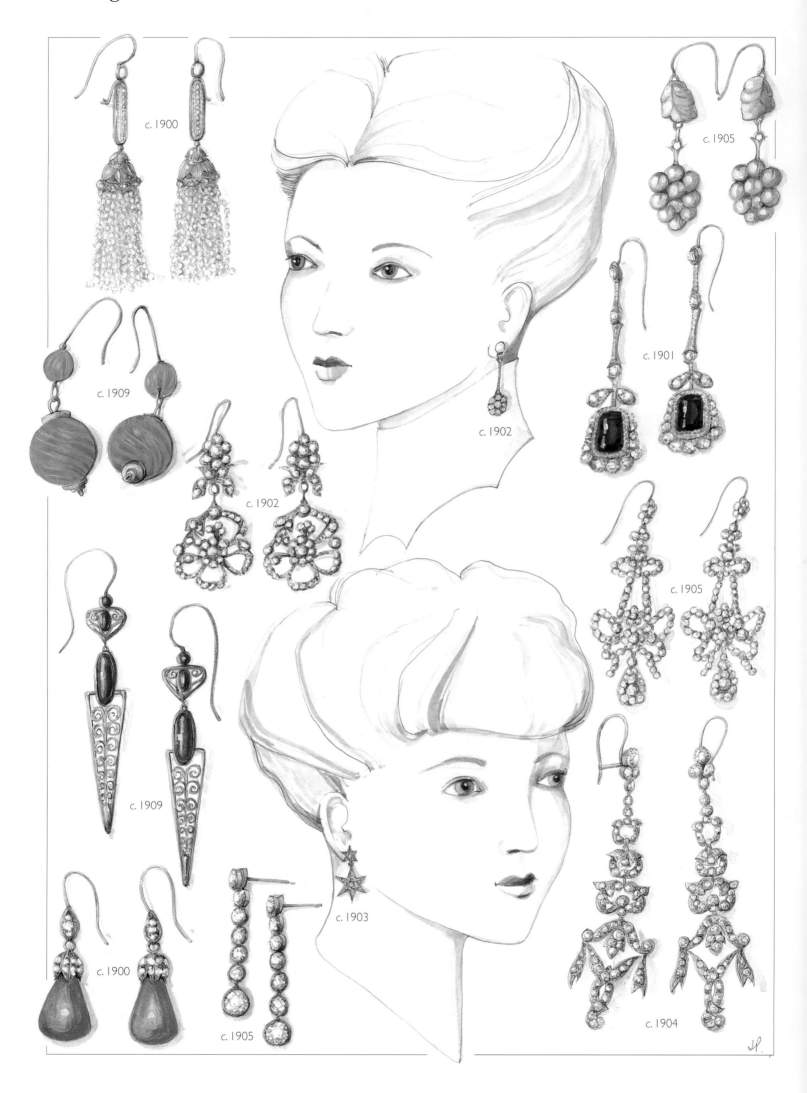

c. 1900

c. 1905

c. 1909

c. 1901

c. 1902

c. 1902

c. 1905

c. 1909

c. 1903

c. 1900

c. 1905

c. 1904

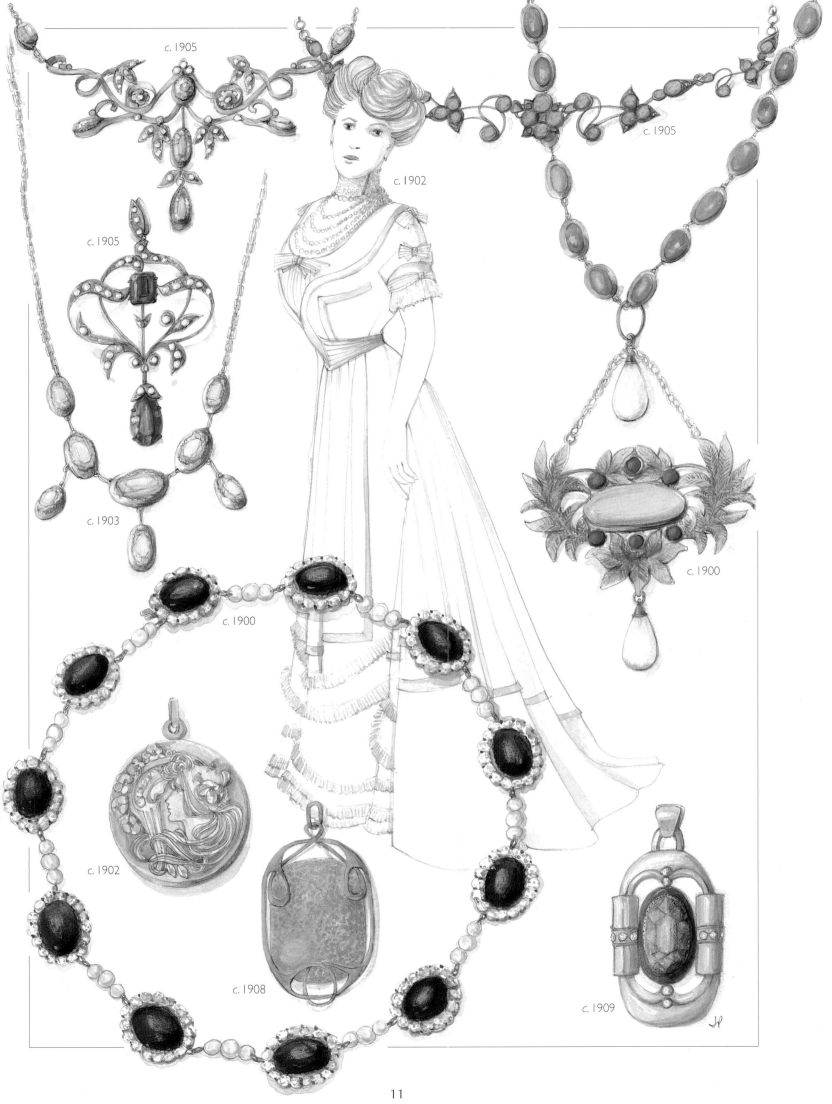

c. 1905

c. 1905

c. 1902

c. 1905

c. 1905

c. 1903

c. 1900

c. 1900

c. 1902

c. 1908

c. 1909

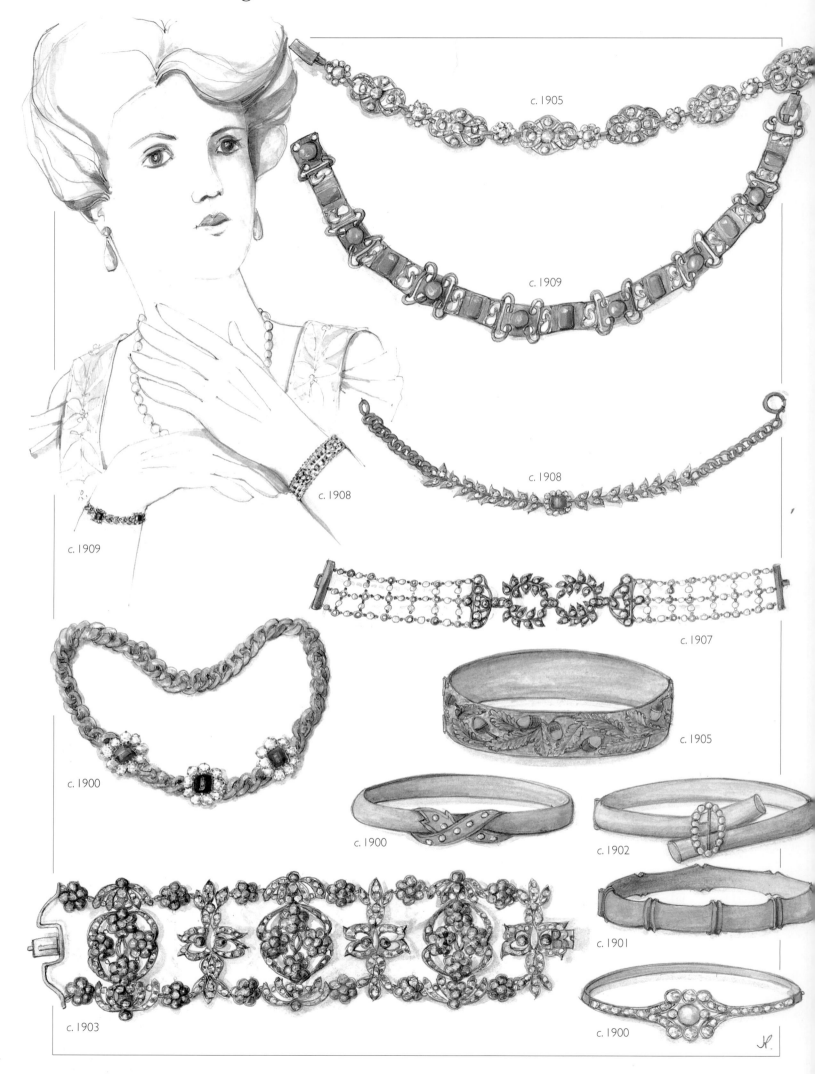

c. 1905

c. 1909

c. 1908

c. 1908

c. 1909

c. 1907

c. 1905

c. 1900

c. 1900

c. 1902

c. 1901

c. 1903

c. 1900

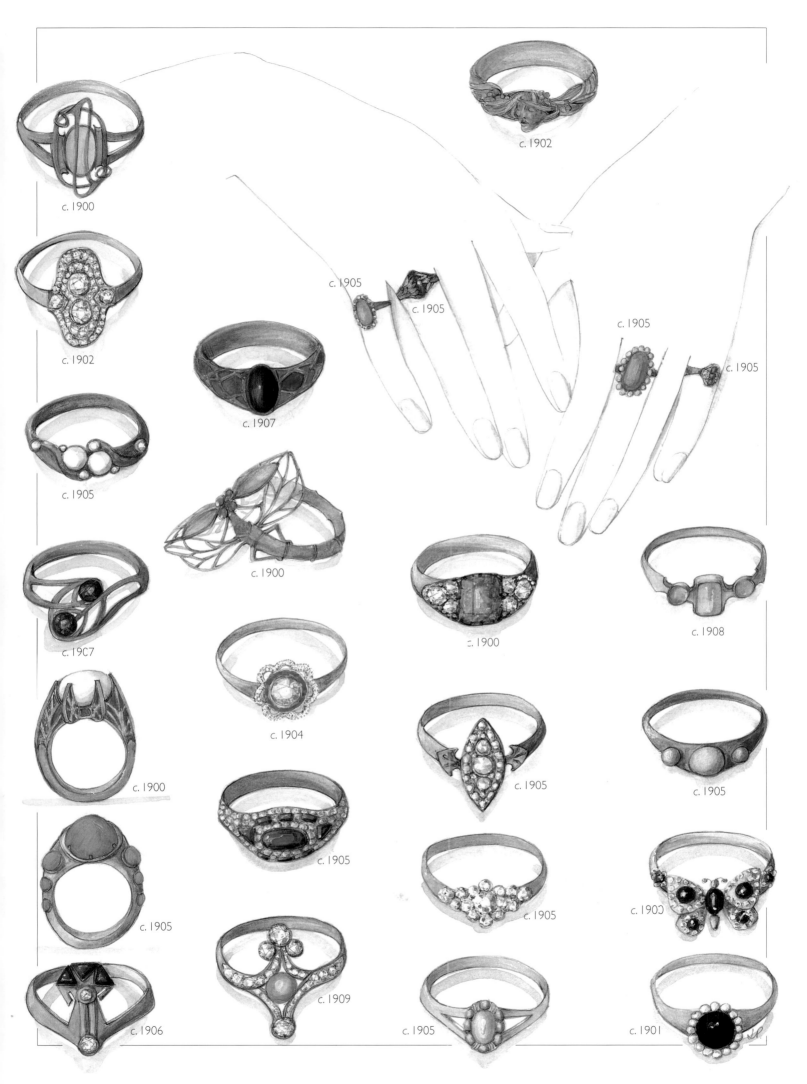

c. 1900

c. 1902

c. 1902

c. 1905

c. 1907

c. 1905

c. 1905

c. 1905

c. 1905

c. 1900

c. 1907

c. 1900

c. 1908

c. 1900

c. 1904

c. 1905

c. 1905

c. 1905

c. 1906

c. 1909

c. 1905

c. 1905

c. 1900

c. 1901

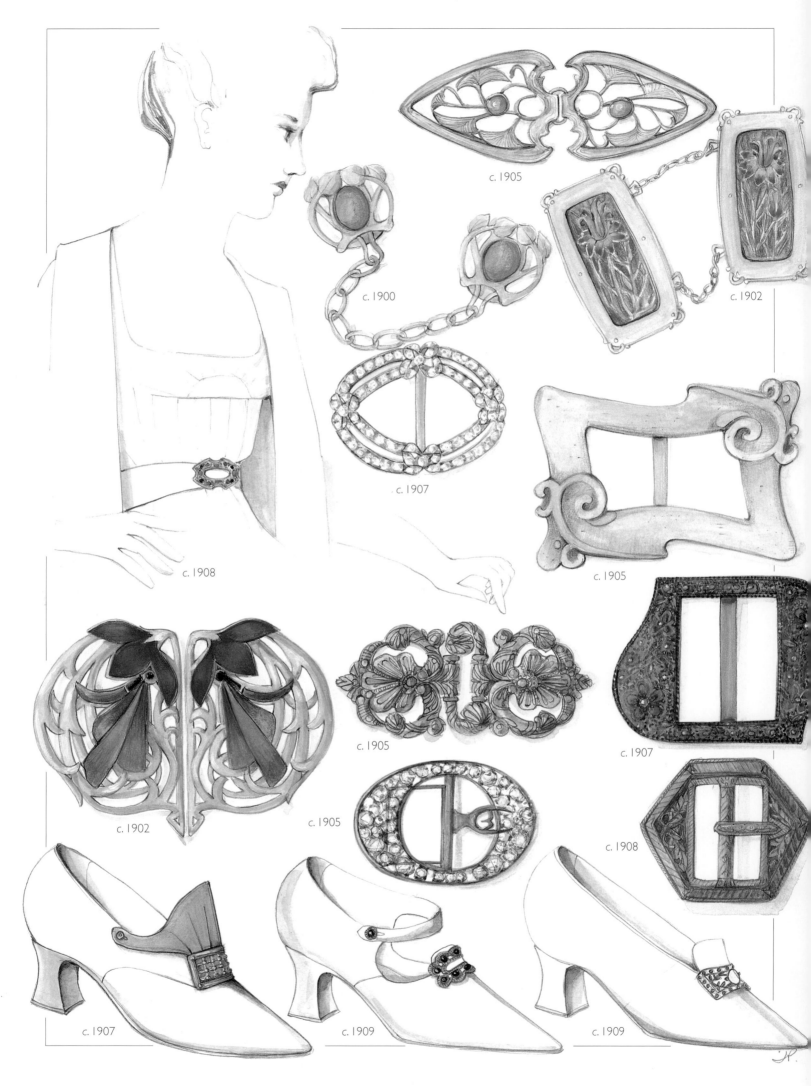

c. 1905

c. 1900

c. 1902

c. 1907

c. 1908

c. 1905

c. 1902

c. 1905

c. 1905

c. 1907

c. 1908

c. 1907

c. 1909

c. 1909

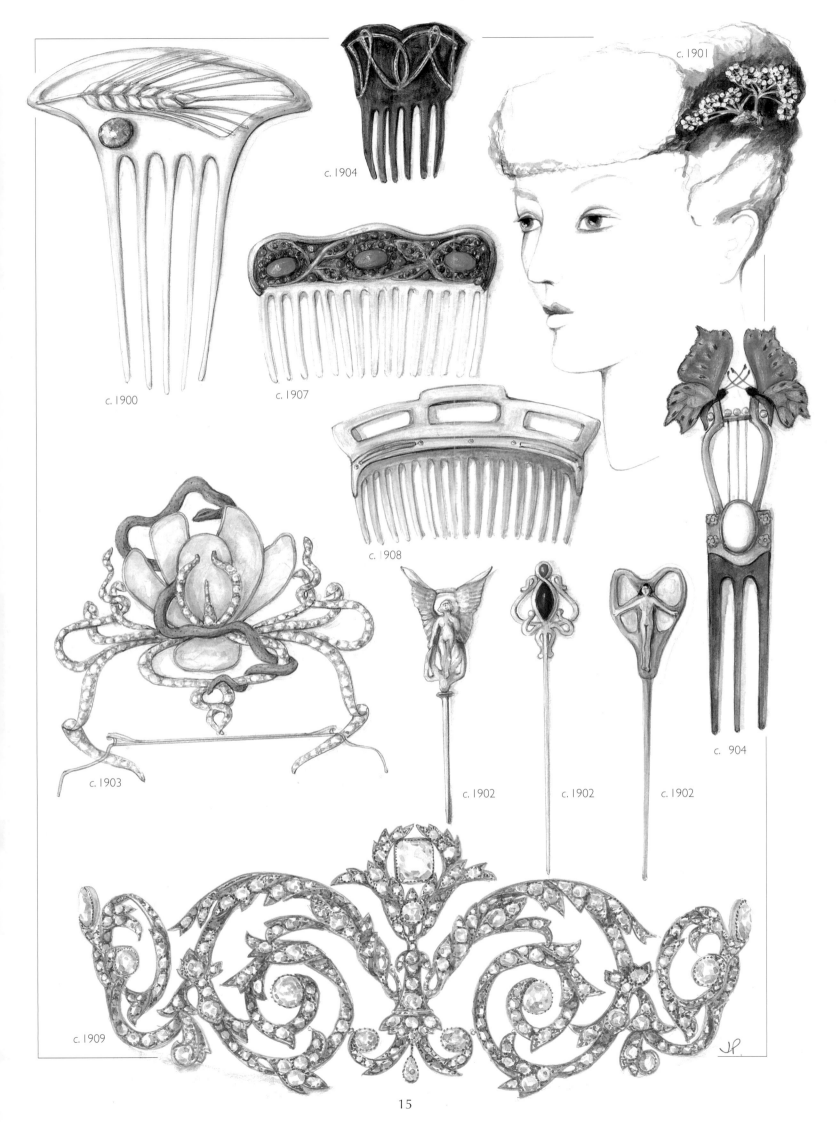

c. 1904

c. 1901

c. 1900

c. 1907

c. 1908

c. 1903

c. 1902

c. 1902

c. 1902

c. 904

c. 1909

Brooches 1910–1919

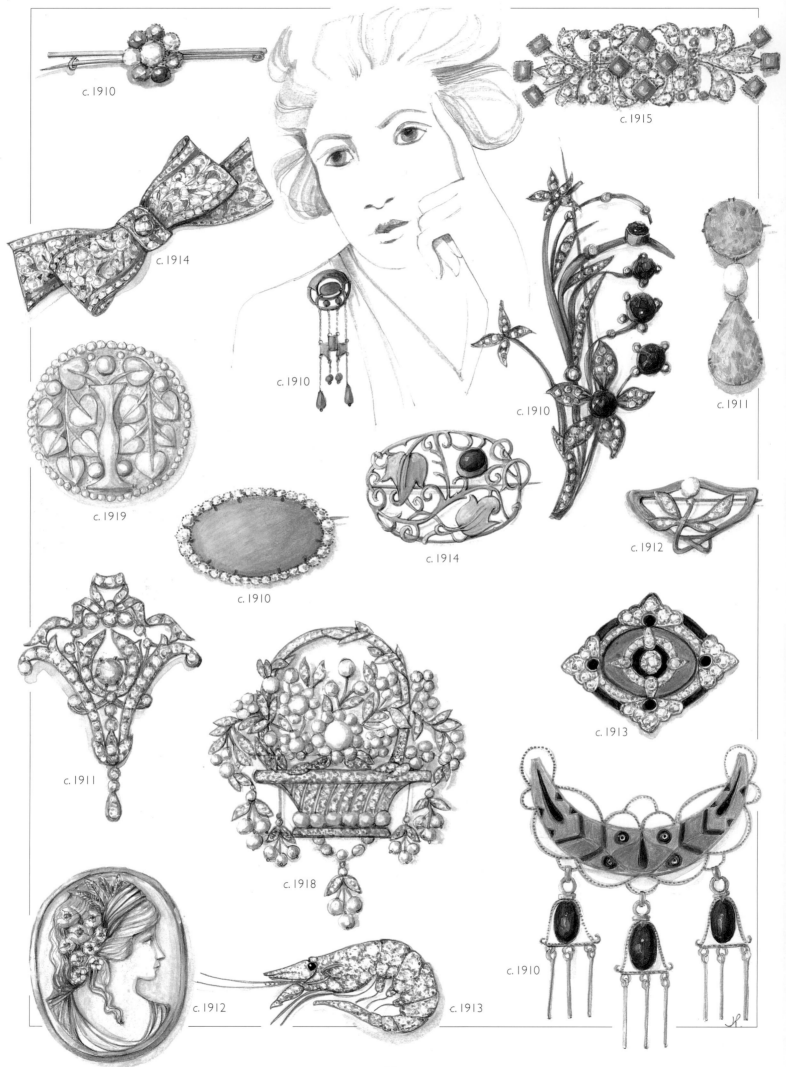

c. 1910

c. 1915

c. 1914

c. 1910

c. 1910

c. 1911

c. 1919

c. 1910

c. 1914

c. 1912

c. 1911

c. 1913

c. 1918

c. 1910

c. 1912

c. 1913

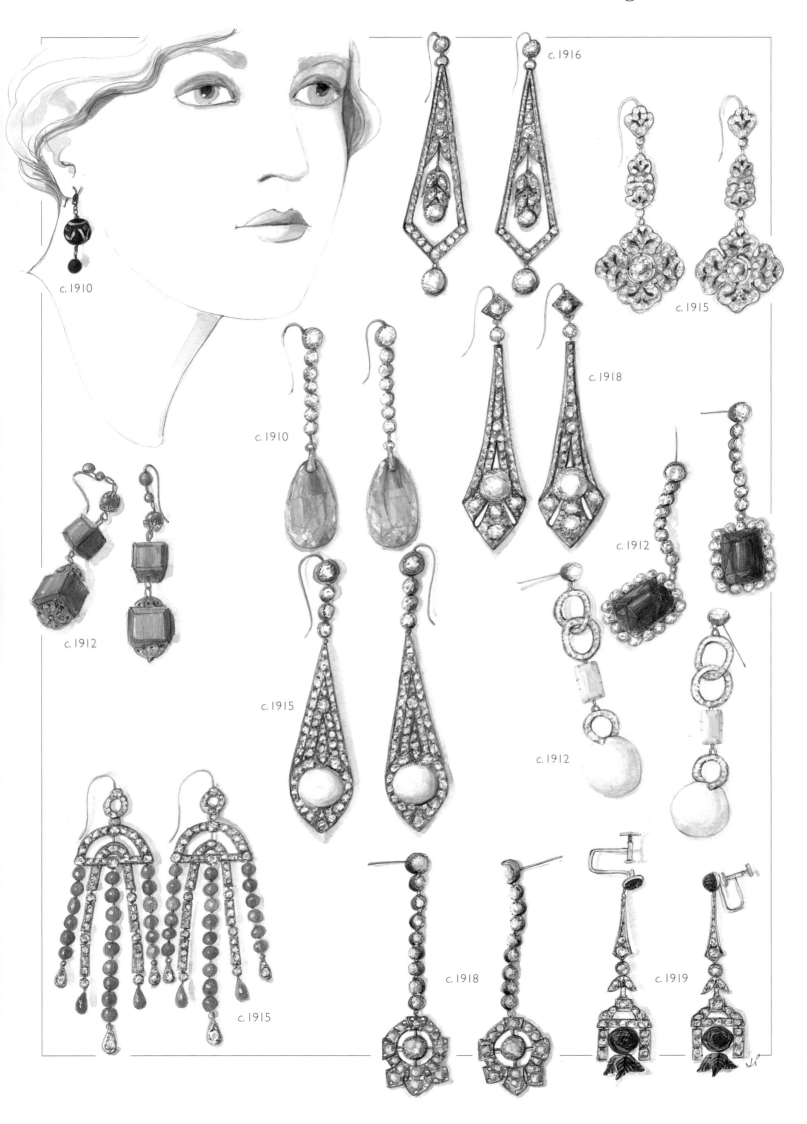

c. 1910

c. 1916

c. 1915

c. 1910

c. 1918

c. 1912

c. 1915

c. 1912

c. 1912

c. 1915

c. 1918

c. 1919

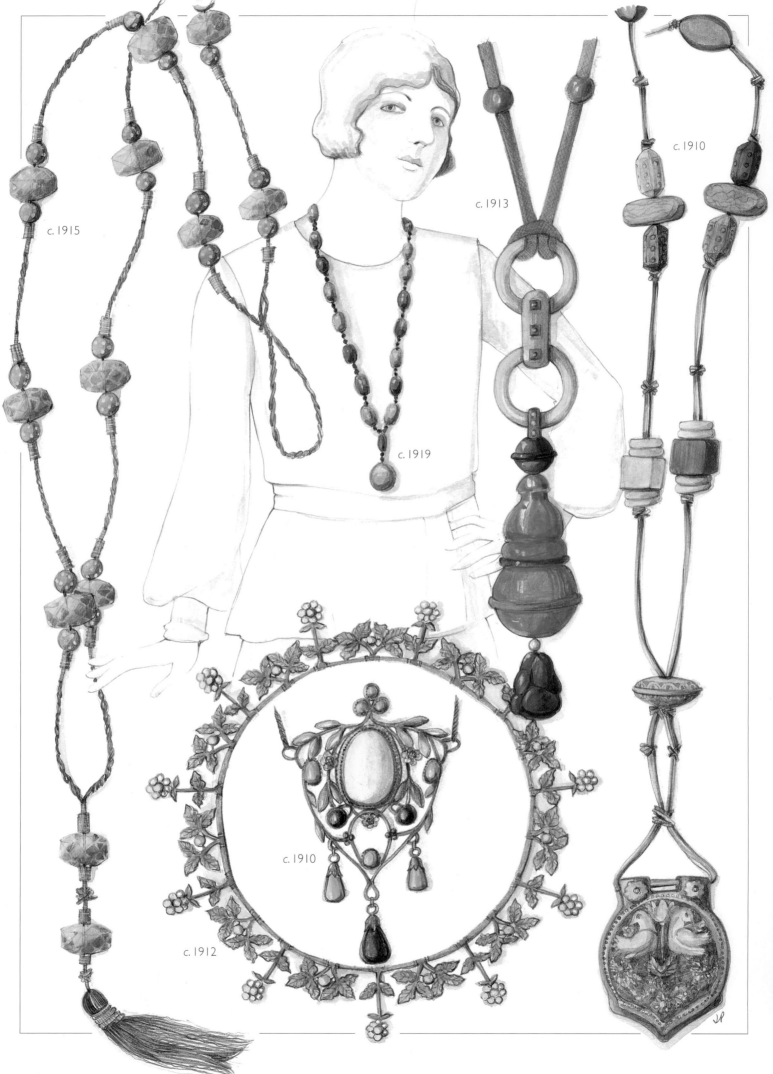

c. 1915

c. 1913

c. 1910

c. 1919

c. 1910

c. 1912

c. 1910

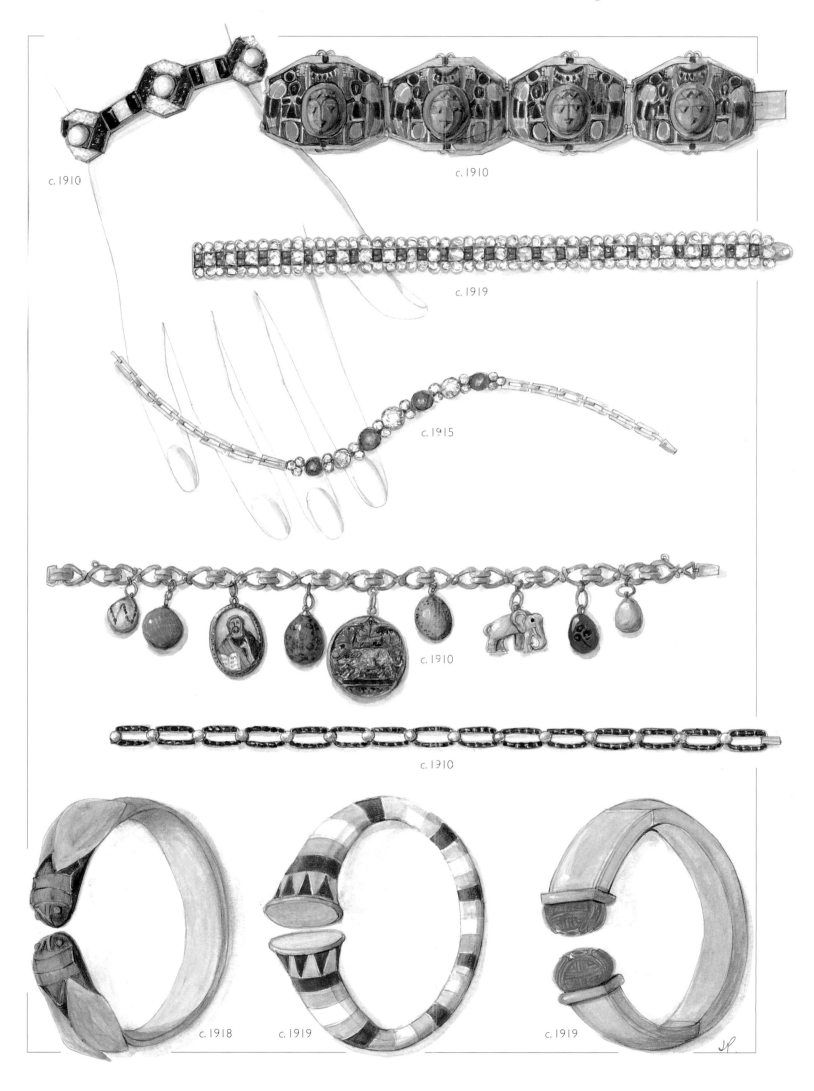

c. 1910

c. 1910

c. 1919

c. 1915

c. 1910

c. 1910

c. 1918

c. 1919

c. 1919

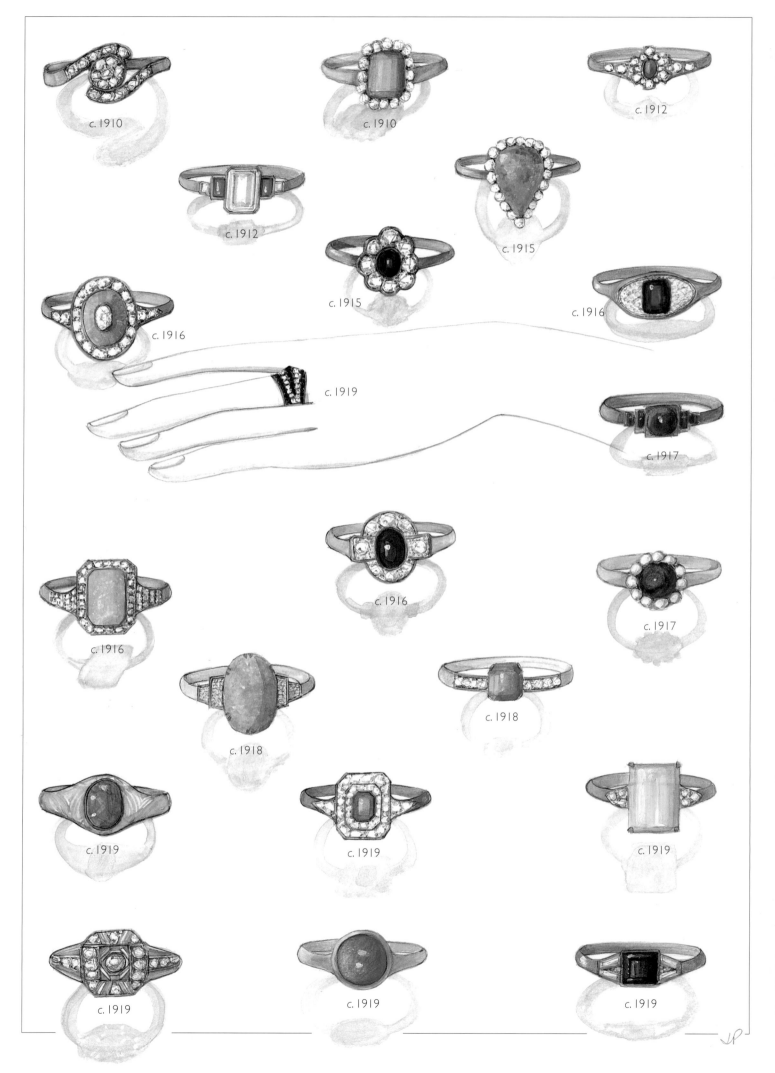

c. 1910

c. 1910

c. 1912

c. 1912

c. 1915

c. 1915

c. 1916

c. 1916

c. 1916

c. 1919

c. 1917

c. 1916

c. 1916

c. 1917

c. 1918

c. 1918

c. 1919

c. 1919

c. 1919

c. 1919

c. 1919

c. 1919

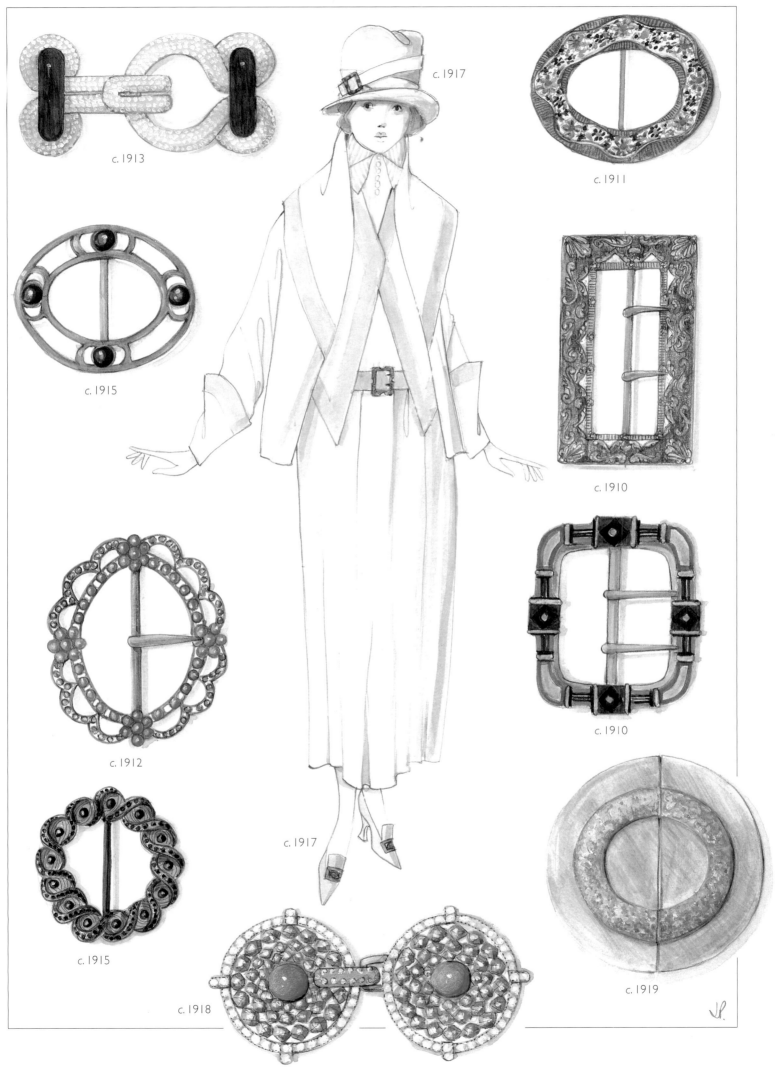

c. 1913

c. 1917

c. 1911

c. 1915

c. 1910

c. 1912

c. 1910

c. 1917

c. 1915

c. 1918

c. 1919

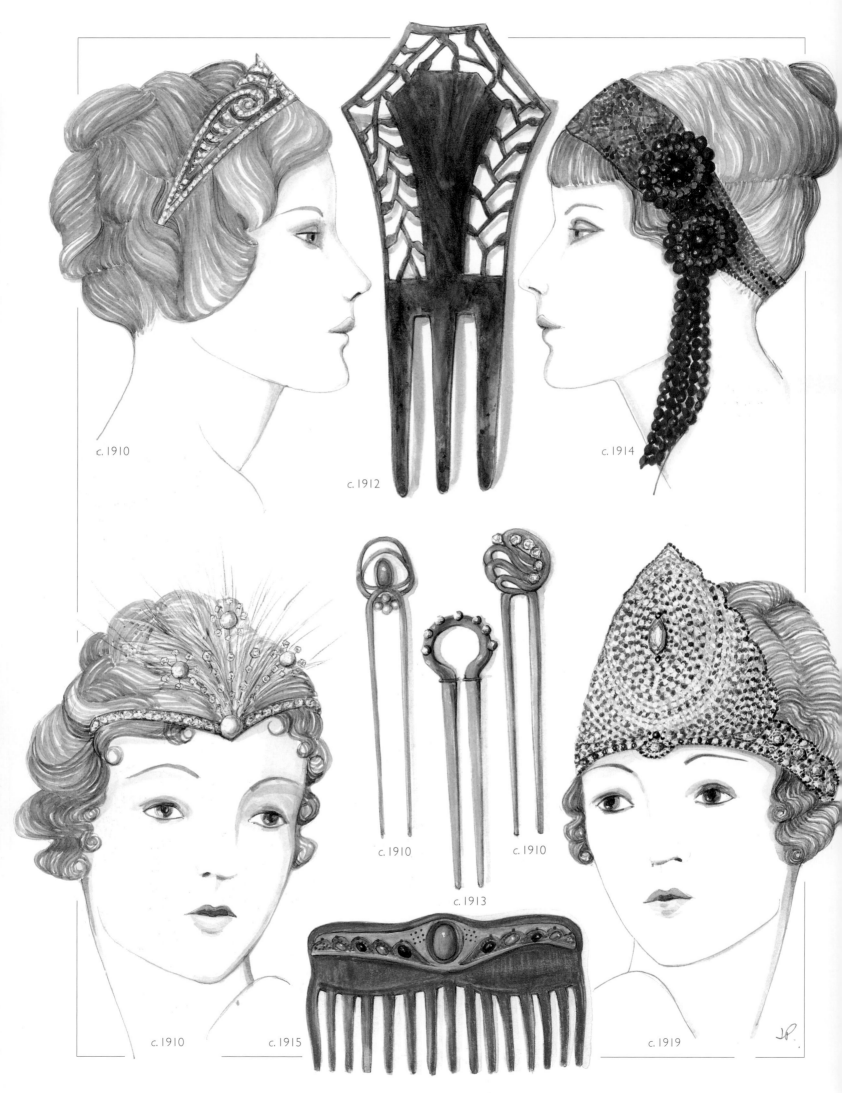

c. 1910

c. 1912

c. 1914

c. 1910

c. 1910

c. 1913

c. 1910

c. 1915

c. 1919

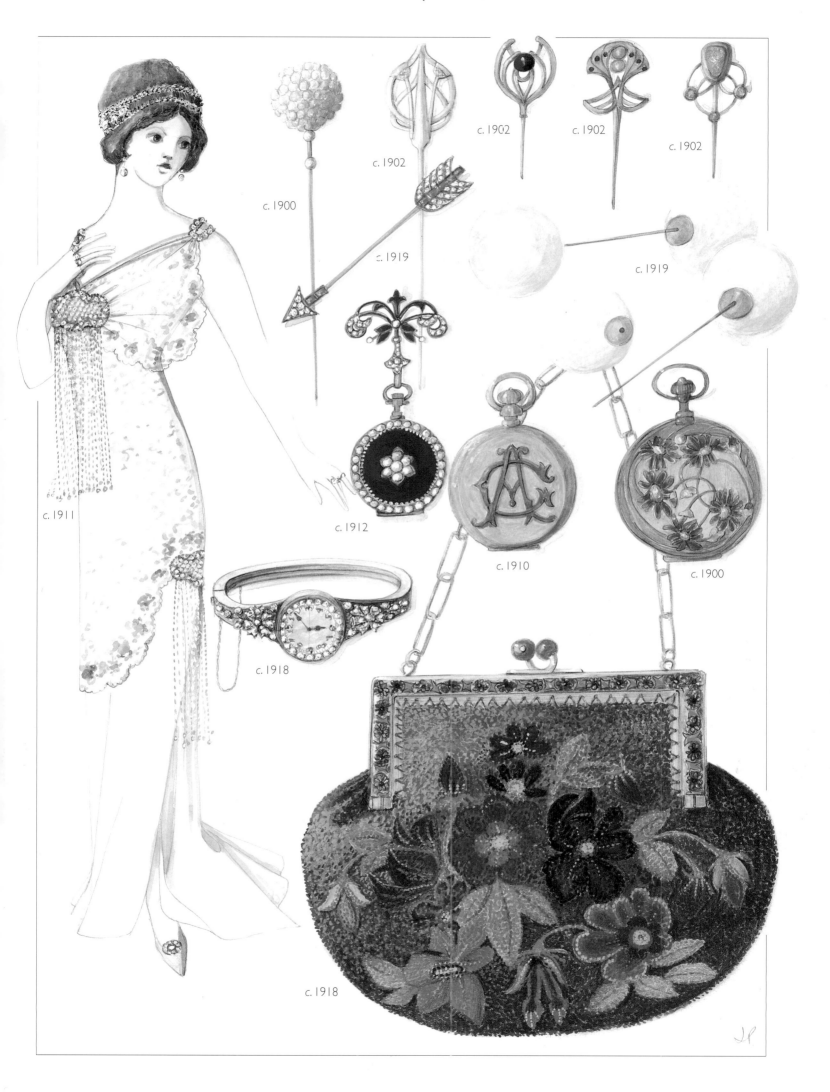

c. 1900

c. 1902

c. 1902

c. 1902

c. 1902

c. 1919

c. 1919

c. 1911

c. 1912

c. 1910

c. 1900

c. 1918

c. 1918

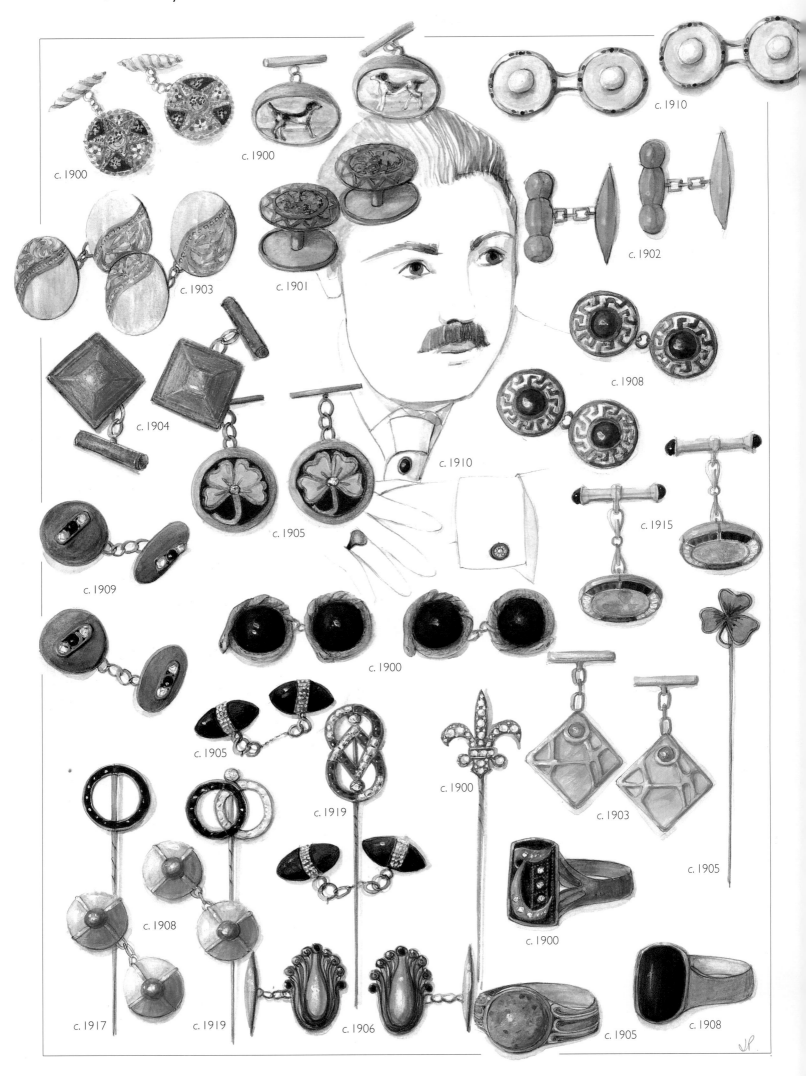

c. 1900

c. 1900

c. 1910

c. 1900

c. 1902

c. 1903

c. 1901

c. 1908

c. 1904

c. 1910

c. 1905

c. 1915

c. 1909

c. 1900

c. 1905

c. 1919

c. 1900

c. 1903

c. 1908

c. 1917

c. 1919

c. 1906

c. 1900

c. 1905

c. 1905

c. 1908

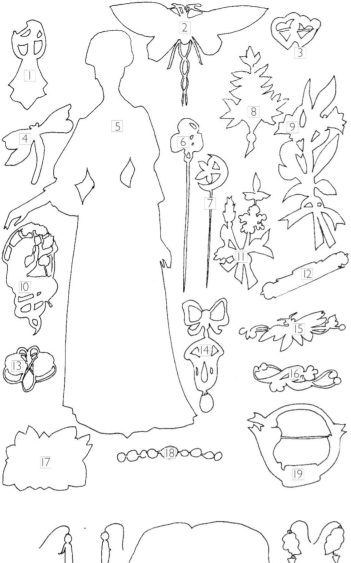

Brooches and Pins 1900–1909

1 c. 1905. Enamelled silver-gilt brooch, floral and foliate design.
2 c. 1900. Yellow celluloid corsage ornament, butterfly design, spot-painted wings, gilt antennae and legs, brooch set with fake pearls and coloured-glass stones. 3 c. 1907. Silver and silver-gilt linked hearts brooch, set with fake pearls and rubies. 4 c. 1905. Enamelled silver brooch, dragonfly design. 5 c. 1907. Silver brooch, lizard design set with fake emeralds, diamonds and rubies. 6 c. 1902. Beaten-silver and enamel lapel pin, abstract design. In the style of David Veasey.
7 c. 1903 Gold lapel pin, crescent and star design, set with pearls.
8 c. 1902. Gold-coloured metal brooch, foliate design, set with clear paste stones. 9 c. 1900. Silver-coloured metal brooch, floral spray, set with coloured and clear paste stones. 10 c. 1902. Silver brooch, mermaid design, enamelled flower heads. In the style of E. May Brown.
11 c. 1908. Gold brooch, floral and foliate design, set with pearls.
12 c. 1900. Polished-brass brooch, set with oval aventurine quartz stone, hollow body to hold needles. 13 c. 1902. Silver-gilt and enamel brooch, foliate and fruit design. In the style of Kate Allen. 14 c. 1905. Gold pendant brooch, set with large turquoise stones and pearls, suspended from bow-shaped pin. In the style of Murrle, Bennett & Co. 15 c. 1904. Silver bar brooch, foliate design with large central fly, pearls set at each end of bar. 16 c. 1909. Gold bar brooch, large central pearl, smaller pearl clusters, twisted bar set with small turquoise stones. 17 c. 1903. Polished-bronze brooch, design of butterfly on bed of leaves. In the style of Mogens Ballin. 18 c. 1900. Gold bar brooch composed of central collet-set emerald, two baroque pearls either side, enamel spacers set with diamonds. 19 c. 1905. Asymmetric silver-gilt brooch, set with graded clear paste stones.

Earrings 1900–1909

1 c. 1900. Gold earrings, studs set with large pearl, pendants set with seed pearls, matching tassels under engraved-gold covers. 2 c. 1905. Silver pendant earrings, design of grapes and leaves. In the style of Georg Jensen. 3 c. 1909. Blown coloured-glass bead earrings, swirling pattern in contrasting colour, silver-gilt links and trim. 4 c. 1902. Silver-gilt earrings, set with colourless rhinestones, floral stud, repeated within pendant wreath. 5 c. 1902. Gold earrings, pearl studs, matching pendants and floral base. 6 c. 1901. Gold and diamond pendant earrings, collet-set ruby encased by diamond borders. In the style of Chaumet. 7 c. 1909. Polished-brass pendant earrings, openwork ribbed-wire head set with large uncut coloured-glass stone, matching pendant link above triangular base. 8 c. 1903. Gold pendant earrings, star-shaped studs set with seed pearls, matching larger base pendants.
9 c. 1905. Silver pendant earrings, set with white paste stones, floral studs, ribbon-bow pendants, floral decoration. 10 c. 1900. Gold earrings, leaf-shaped studs set with diamonds, matching caps above teardrop, polished-emerald pendants. 11 c. 1905. Gold pendant earrings, stud set with brilliant-cut diamond above flexible line of similar stones, ending with large stone. 12 c. 1904. Long silver-gilt earrings, studs set with three large colourless paste stones, flexible pendants in the form of wreaths and garlands set with similar stones.

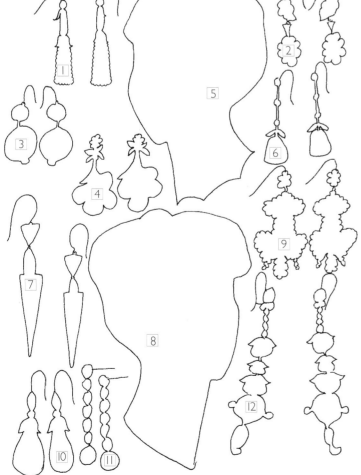

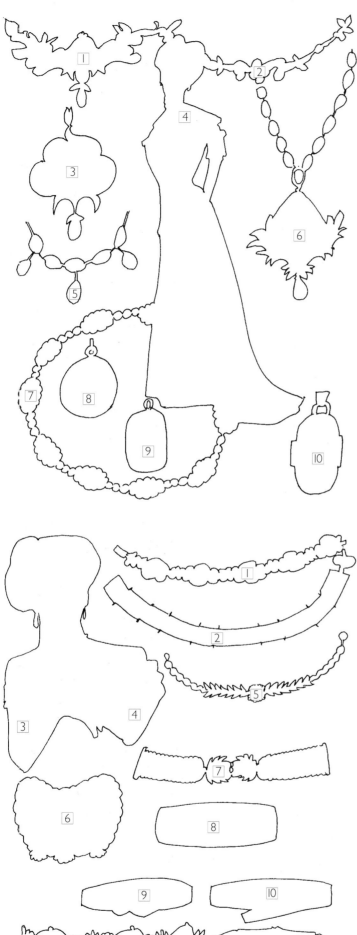

Necklaces and Pendants 1900–1909

1 *c.* 1905. Gold necklace, scrolling mounts set with circular and oval peridots, matching pear-shaped pendant drop, floral and foliate motifs set with half pearls, fine linked back chain. 2 *c.* 1905. Gold necklace, floral and foliate scroll design, set with opals and small garnets, linked chain back. 3 *c.* 1905. Gold pendant, asymmetric scroll design, set with half pearls, central cushion-shaped sapphire, matching pear-shaped pendant drop. 4 *c.* 1902. Deep choker pearl necklace, support bars set with diamonds, worn in conjunction with five-strand pearl necklace, back fastening. 5 *c.* 1903. Pale transparent blue moulded-glass stone necklace set in silver, three pendant drops, linked chain back. 6 *c.* 1900. Opal pendant set in gold, enamel wreath set with sapphire cabochon collets, opal pipkin drop above and below, on a gold necklace set with a line of opals. 7 *c.* 1900. Necklace composed of eleven uniform-size amethyst cabochon and diamond oval-shaped clusters mounted in gold and silver collets and divided by triple pearl spacers, invisible clasp fastening. 8 *c.* 1902. Gold-coloured pendant, front modelled with female bust profile, swivel action reveals two mirrors. 9 *c.* 1908. Large turquoise set in gold scroll mount. In the style of Murrle, Bennett & Co. 10 *c.* 1909. Polished-metal pendant, vertical sided bars banded and set with white paste stones, centrally mounted large moulded-glass stone.

Bracelets and Bangles 1900–1909

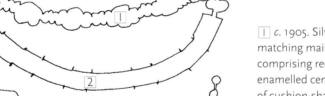

1 *c.* 1905. Silver-gilt bracelet, floral links set with white paste stones, matching main ribbon-bow-shaped pieces. 2 *c.* 1909. Gold bracelet comprising rectangular plates set either with turquoise stone or enamelled centre, pierced sides, linked wire rings. 3 *c.* 1909. Bracelet of cushion-shaped rubies with diamond surround, foliate spacers set with diamonds. 4 *c.* 1908. Wide gold bracelet, pierced design, set with diamonds, rubies and pearls. 5 *c.* 1908. Silver-gilt bracelet, flexible foliate links set with white paste stones either side cushion-shaped fake emerald with white paste stone surround, linked chain back. 6 *c.* 1900. Gold bracelet, three diamond and gem clusters, ruby, sapphire and emerald centres mounted on a plain curb link chain. In the style of Tiffany & Co. 7 *c.* 1907. Gold bracelet, two foliate central wreaths set with diamonds, matching side bars attaching linked pearl and gold chain sides to clasp fastening. 8 *c.* 1905. Two-piece hinged gold bangle, acorn and oakleaf enamelled design, engraved background. 9 *c.* 1900. Narrow gold bangle, opening under pearl-set knot on centre front. 10 *c.* 1902. Narrow hinged gold bangle, crossover on centre front, pearl-set oval buckle. 11 *c.* 1903. Wide silver bracelet, floral garlands and ribbon bows set with white and coloured paste stones. 12 *c.* 1901. Hinged gold bangle, bamboo design. 13 *c.* 1900. Narrow bangle, pearl set within diamond surround, matching shoulders, plain gold back.

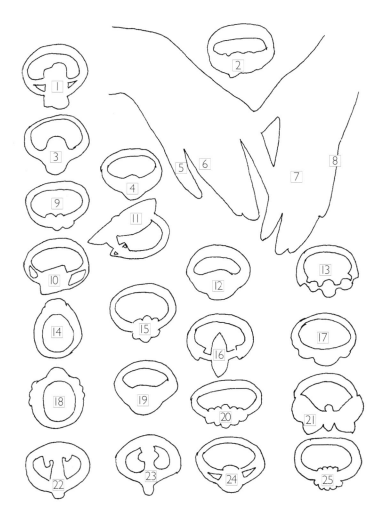

Rings 1900–1909

1 *c.* 1900. Flat stone set under complex frame. In the style of Archibald Knox. 2 *c.* 1902. Modelled head, hair intertwined with leaves and berries on gold band. 3 *c.* 1902. Two large diamonds, diamond surround set in platinum. 4 *c.* 1907. Enamelled shaped gold band, oval cabochon ruby. 5 *c.* 1905. Oval turquoise, diamond surround set in gold. 6 *c.* 1905. Engraved-gold band, red stone. 7 *c.* 1905. Large oval cabochon emerald, pearl surround, set in gold. 8 *c.* 1905. Silver ring set with green stones in vertical row. 9 *c.* 1905. Graded pearls set in gold band. 10 *c.* 1907. Gold ring, pierced frame set with two rubies. 11 *c.* 1900. Gold dragonfly ring set with opals. In the style of René Lalique. 12 *c.* 1900. Claw-set central paste stone, three-stone shoulders. 13 *c.* 1908. Oblong cabochon stone, round cabochon stone on each shoulder. 14 *c.* 1900. Enamelled foliate design, pearl setting. In the style of René Lalique. 15 *c.* 1904. Large diamond, emerald surround, pierced and scalloped border. 16 *c.* 1905. Shield-shaped ring set with diamonds, foliate shoulders. 17 *c.* 1905. Gold band set with three black pearls. 18 *c.* 1905. Central cabochon turquoise, matching stones on shoulders. 19 *c.* 1905. Cabochon oval sapphire, diamond and sapphire surround, diamond shoulders. 20 *c.* 1905. Gold band, central cluster of diamonds. 21 *c.* 1900. Gold butterfly set with diamonds and rubies. 22 *c.* 1906. Flat gold wire ring set with diamonds and rubies. 23 *c.* 1909. Pink pearl set within pierced surround of diamonds. 24 *c.* 1905. Central chalcedony stone, carved silver surround, pierced shoulders. In the style of Georg Jensen. 25 *c.* 1901. Round cabochon ruby, pearl surround.

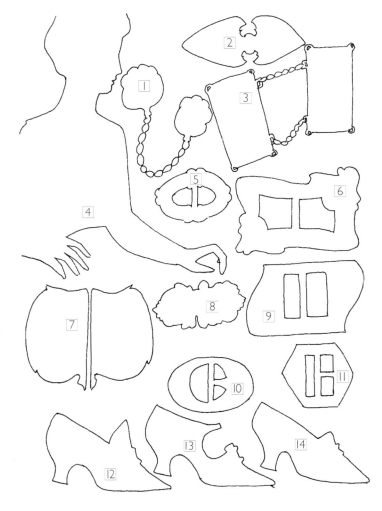

Buckles and Clasps 1900–1909

1 *c.* 1900. Beaten-silver cloak clasps, openwork foliate-design brooches set with large blue stones, linked silver chain. 2 *c.* 1905. Gold-coloured metal belt clasps with spear-shaped plates, Egyptian-revival design of lotus flowers against a pierced background, set with coloured-glass stones. 3 *c.* 1902. Wrought-silver cape clasps, panels of enamelled flowers two silver link chains. In the style of Nelson and Edith Dawson. 4 *c.* 1908. Gold-coloured metal belt-buckle, cut edges, set with multicoloured glass stones. 5 *c.* 1907. Oval silver-gilt belt-buckle, two bands set with white paste stones, joined in four places by tied bows. 6 *c.* 1905. Beaten-silver belt-buckle, curved edges, scroll decoration on two corners. 7 *c.* 1902. Pierced-silver belt clasp, enamelled flower and insect decoration. In the style of Annie Alabaster. 8 *c.* 1905. Cast-bronze belt clasp, stylized foliate-design matching plates. 9 *c.* 1907. Bronze and gold-coloured celluloid belt-buckle, design of flowers and scattered beads, curved asymmetric sides. 10 *c.* 1905. Oval gilt evening shoe buckle set with white paste stones. 11 *c.* 1908. Daywear metal shoe-buckle, engraved design, mock pin. 12 *c.* 1907. Two-tone leather shoes, gold-coloured metal shoe-buckle, central mesh panel. 13 *c.* 1909. Satin evening shoes, ribbed-wire shoe-buckles set with coloured-glass stones, matching buttons on bar straps. 14 *c.* 1909. Patent-leather shoes, short tongues, black openwork steel buckle.

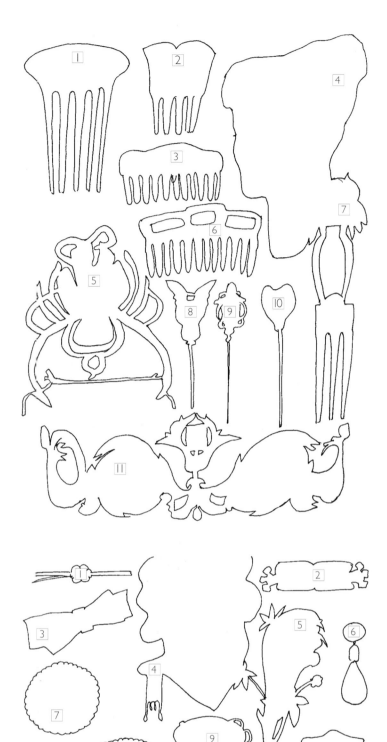

Hair Ornaments, Combs and Pins 1900–1909

1 *c.* 1900. Carved horn haircomb, single amber stone, carved and pierced wheatsheaf motif. In the style of Lucien Gaillard. 2 *c.* 1904. Mock-tortoiseshell celluloid haircomb, inset silver loop and scallop design. 3 *c.* 1907. Ivory haircomb, engraved-silver mount set with coloured stones. 4 *c.* 1901. Carved hair ornament, stylized cow parsley design. In the style of Lucien Gaillard. 5 *c.* 1903. Gold hair ornament, set with diamonds, central flower motif of opals, textured gold serpent. In the style of Philippe Wolfers. 6 *c.* 1908. Tortoiseshell haircomb, pierced silver mount. 7 *c.* 1904. Tortoiseshell haircomb, gold mount set with large fake pearl, lyre-shaped top with two facing enamelled butterflies, small fake pearl trim. 8 *c.* 1902. Silver hairpin, angel design, wings touched with enamel. In the style of Annie McLeish. 9 *c.* 1902. Silver hairpin, pierced scrollwork, enamelled panels emulating stones. In the style of E. M. Hodgkinson. 10 *c.* 1902. Gold hairpin, fairy design, enamelled figure, mother-of-pearl set with wings. In the style of W. Hodgkinson. 11 *c.* 1909. Gold and silver tiara, running scrollwork design, set with various sized diamonds. In the style of Chaumet.

Brooches 1910–1919

1 *c.* 1910. Gold bar brooch, set with fancy colour diamonds in central floral design. 2 *c.* 1915. Gold brooch, fleur-de-lys design, set with emeralds and diamonds. 3 *c.* 1914. Platinum brooch, waved bow, pierced scroll design set with diamonds, highlighted with lines of emeralds, central knot set with large diamond. 4 *c.* 1910. Pierced-silver brooch, set with blue and green stones, matching beads on ends of pendant chains. 5 *c.* 1910. Silver-coloured metal brooch, flower spray set with paste stones. 6 *c.* 1911. Circular aquamarine brooch, claw set in gold, matching teardrop, spaced by baroque pearl. 7 *c.* 1919. Round grained silver brooch, vase and leaf design, polished-bead edge. 8 *c.* 1910. Oval green stone mounted in silver, graduated surround of white paste stones. 9 *c.* 1914. Oval silver brooch, pierced background of tendrils and leaves, single asymmetric cabochon stone. 10 *c.* 1912. Gold brooch, wing-shaped frame, open centre linked by four diamond-set leaves and single pearl and diamond flower. 11 *c.* 1911. Scroll-and-ribbon brooch, set with diamonds, single central yellow diamond. 12 *c.* 1918. Corsage brooch, gold set with diamonds and pearls, basket of fruit and flowers. In the style of Cartier. 13 *c.* 1913. Oval black plastic-onyx brooch, set with white paste stones, plastic-jade inset. Copy in the style of Cartier. 14 *c.* 1912. Moulded opaque glass cameo, highlights of red paint, set in gold metal frame. 15 *c.* 1913. Gold shrimp brooch, set with diamonds, ruby eye. In the style of Cartier. 16 *c.* 1910. Half-moon-shaped gilded-silver brooch, multicoloured enamel, wire frame, amethyst pendants. In the style of Adolf Hildenbrand.

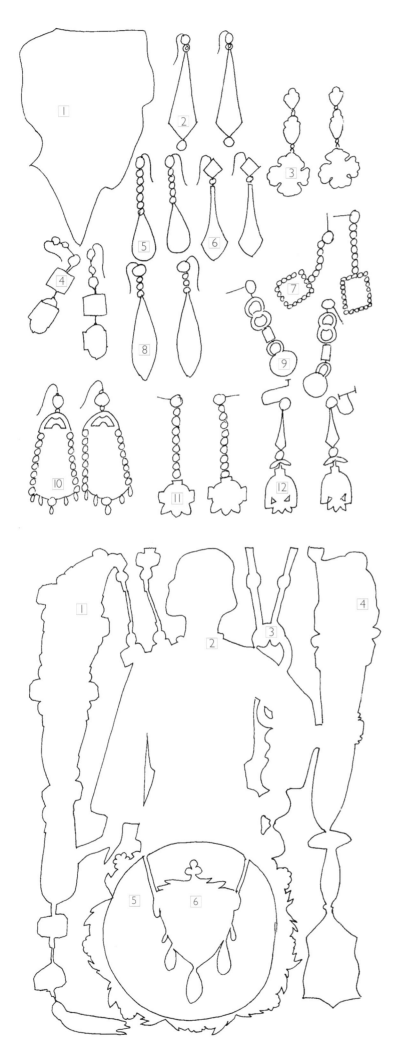

Earrings 1910–1919

1 c. 1910. Moulded coloured-glass pendant earrings, large ball multicoloured raised glass pattern suspended from fine gold chain, matching small undecorated ball below, gold fixings. 2 c. 1916. Platinum pierced kite-shaped earrings set with diamonds, matching suspended foliate detail, large diamond pendant. 3 c. 1915. Platinum and gold pendant earrings, foliate and floral design set with diamonds. 4 c. 1912. Plastic imitation-amber pendant earrings, two cubes with silver-gilt trim, chain links, matching small bead under gold bead studs. 5 c. 1910. Large aquamarine pendant drop suspended under row of graded millegrain-set diamonds, gold fixings. 6 c. 1918. Platinum pierced kite-shaped pendant earrings, set with large central diamond surrounded by similar diamonds. 7 c. 1912. Cushion-shaped synthetic amethysts, diamond surround, suspended from row of matching diamonds. 8 c. 1915. Platinum and gold earrings, long teardrop pendants set with large fake pearls surrounded by diamonds, suspended from line of matching stones. 9 c. 1912. Gold pendant earrings, cushion-shaped sapphire between diamond-set links above large pearl. 10 c. 1915. Gold pendant earrings, set with diamonds, matching links between rows of jade beads, finishing alternate diamond and jade drops. 11 c. 1918. Silver-gilt earrings paste-peridot floral pendants suspended below row of matching stones. 12 c. 1919. Silver pendant earrings set with clear paste stones and moulded coloured-glass flowers and leaves, adjustable screw fastenings.

Sautoirs, Necklaces and Pendants 1910–1919

1 c. 1915. Fine twisted silk sautoir, moulded coloured-glass beads spaced by smaller glass beads patterned with raised contrast-colour spots bound in place by gold wire, matching pendant ending in a long silk tassel. 2 c. 1919. Waist-length sautoir, painted multicoloured flat stone oval beads, spaced by small black beads, matching pendant ending in a large flat painted disc. 3 c. 1913. Glass and plastic pendant, plastic rings linked by fake sapphire-studded bar, matching small bar supporting fake ruby and large carved coloured-glass pear-shaped stone, above fake pearl and small carved coloured-glass stone drop. Tubular knitted-silk cord back. Imitating the style of Cartier. 4 c. 1910. Multicoloured knotted-silk-cord sautoir threaded with various sized and multicoloured carved wooden beads and discs, large shield-shaped gold painted carved wood pendant, design of birds, fruit and flowers. 5 c. 1912. Fine gold necklace, foliate and floral design gilded and touched with coloured enamels, spaced by small pink pearls, matching pearl flowers. In the style of Georges Fouquet. 6 c. 1910. Silver pendant, large central coloured stone, floral and foliate background set with small coloured stones and drops, pendant suspended from silk cord. In the style of Arthur and Georgina Gaskin.

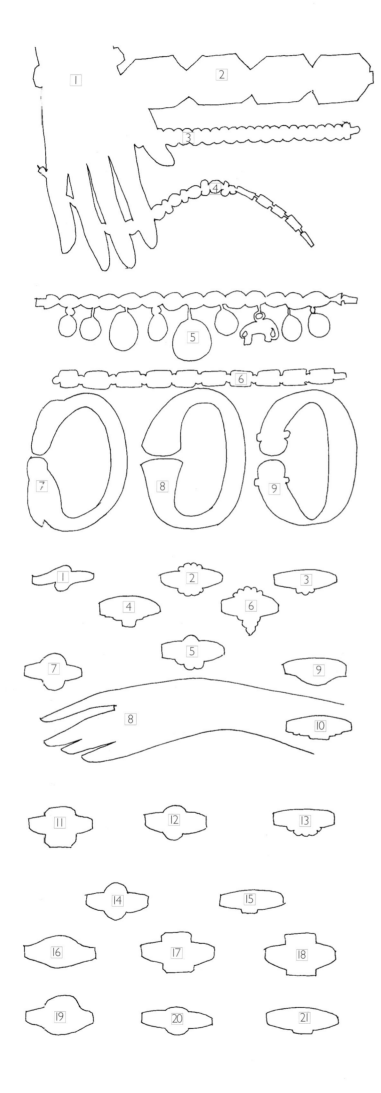

Bracelets and Bangles 1910–1919

1 *c.* 1910. Gold bracelet, hexagonal motifs, each set with large central pearl, diamond and ruby surround, onyx and diamond links. 2 *c.* 1910. Egyptian-revival-style silver bracelet, hinged plates decorated with multicoloured enamels, set with coloured stones, central carved stone portrait. 3 *c.* 1919. Platinum bracelet, set in a line of uniform brilliants and pairs of square-cut synthetic sapphires vertically set between. Flanked by diamond collets in arched borders. 4 *c.* 1915. Sapphire and diamond bracelet, collet-set, three brilliant-cut diamonds and four circular sapphires, smaller brilliants set between, white-gold brick-link back. 5 *c.* 1910. Russian charm bracelet, nine charms, including miniature gold elephant with ruby eyes; circular medallion depicting a wild boar; gold and red enamel egg pendant, set with a trefoil cluster of rubies. 6 *c.* 1910. Narrow pierced-gold band bracelet, comprising oblong fake ruby and onyx links between alternate pink and grey imitation pearls. 7 *c.* 1918. Open plastic bangle, facing large painted winged insects. 8 *c.* 1919. Egyptian-revival-style fake-ivory bangle, painted in broad bands of colour through to flared opening. 9 *c.* 1919. Ivory bangle, deep silver mounts and carved jade beads at each side of opening.

Rings 1910–1919

1 *c.* 1910. Ring set with floral cluster of diamonds, diamond-set scroll shoulders. 2 *c.* 1910. Cushion-shaped emerald, diamond surround. 3 *c.* 1912. Central oval emerald, diamond surround, diamond-set shoulders. 4 *c.* 1912. Central cushion-shaped clear paste stone, matching paste and fake sapphire shoulders. 5 *c.* 1915. Synthetic ruby, diamond surround. 6 *c.* 1915. Large pear-shaped opal, white paste stone surround. 7 *c.* 1916. Centrally set diamond, pavé-set emerald inner surround, diamond surround, matching shoulders. 8 *c.* 1919. Deep flared band, pavé-set rows of rubies and diamonds. 9 *c.* 1916. Boat-shaped mount set with cushion-shaped sapphire, pavé-set diamond surround, shaped shoulders. 10 *c.* 1917. Centrally set half glass bead on square mount, stepped shoulders set with matching stones. 11 *c.* 1916. Large cushion-shaped opal set within octagonal mount of diamonds, matching shoulders. 12 *c.* 1916. Oval cabochon stone, white paste surround and shoulders. 13 *c.* 1917. Black pearl, white pearl surround. 14 *c.* 1918. Oval opal, diamond-set stepped shoulders. 15 *c.* 1918. Cushion-shaped emerald, diamond-set shoulders. 16 *c.* 1919. Engraved-silver ring set with cabochon stone. 17 *c.* 1919. Cushion-shaped emerald, double surround of diamonds, matching shoulders. 18 *c.* 1919. Large square aquamarine set between diamond-set shoulders. 19 *c.* 1919. Engraved and pierced ring set with white paste stones. 20 *c.* 1919. Circular hardstone in plain mounts. In the style of Georg Jensen. 21 *c.* 1919. Cushion-shaped ruby, diamond shoulders.

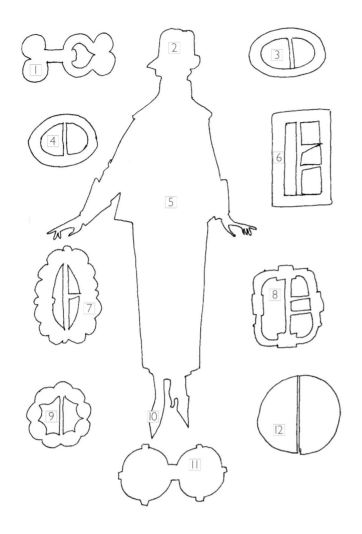

Buckles and Clasps 1910–1919

1 c. 1913. Metal belt clasp in the form of a hook and eye, set with diamanté, bars of polished fake onyx to emulate stitches. 2 c. 1917. Polished silver-gilt hat-buckle set with coloured-glass stones. 3 c. 1911. Oval metal belt-buckle, floral decoration in multicoloured enamels. 4 c. 1915. Oval polished-brass shoe-buckle, pierced and set with four coloured-glass half-beads. 5 c. 1917. Polished-brass belt-buckle, engraved design, cut edges, two-prong fastening. 6 c. 1910. Oblong silver belt-buckle, engraved, raised and pierced design, two-prong fastening. 7 c. 1912. Oval polished-brass belt-buckle, raised and pierced design, scalloped edges between floral detail. 8 c. 1910. Egyptian-revival-style metal belt-buckle, oblong shape with rounded edges, multicoloured enamelled geometric pattern, two-prong fastening. 9 c. 1915. Round engraved-copper shoe-buckle, raised serpentine design around engraved central panels. 10 c. 1917. Silver-gilt shoe-buckles, multicoloured enamelled raised centre plates. 11 c. 1918. Silver-plated metal fur clasp, two matching round plates, centrally set large fake cabochon emerald, graded surround of angular polished beads, outer diamanté surround. 12 c. 1919. Large smooth yellow plastic belt clasp, flat split circular plate with inner circle of blue textured plastic.

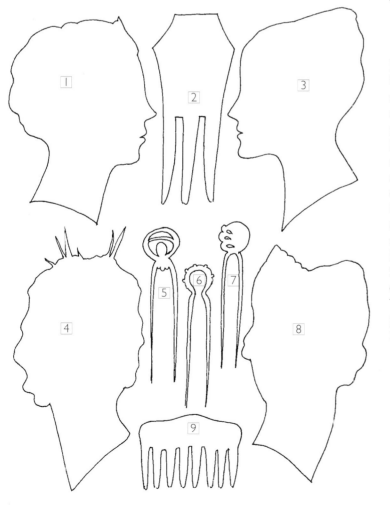

Hair Ornaments 1910–1919

1 c. 1910. Gold bandeau, scroll and foliate design, collet-set diamonds, fine wire supports. 2 c. 1912. Handcarved faux-tortoiseshell haircomb, solid central panel, pierced border, three prongs. 3 c. 1914. Stiffened-silk bandeau, multicoloured leaf design of fine glass beads, two large pink glass-bead motifs worn at one side, adjacent to each other, the lower with shoulder-length bead tassel. 4 c. 1910. Narrow gold and silver aigrette, large pearl above centre front V-shaped peak, diamonds and pearl-and-diamond flower motifs mounted on fine wires among osprey feathers. In the style of Chaumet. 5 c. 1910. Gold wire hairpin, looped wire head set with cabochon sapphire, cluster of gold beads above two prongs. 6 c. 1913. Silver-gilt hairpin, head set with row of seed pearls, two prongs. 7 c. 1910. Polished-brass hairpin, twisted wire head set with row of colourless paste stones, two prongs. 8 c. 1919. Stiffened-silk bandeau, wired scalloped edge, high on centre front, embroidered all over in black, white and silver glass beads. 9 c. 1915. Tortoiseshell haircomb, shaped pierced gold mount set with large central pale amethyst, matching smaller two-colour stones within scroll design. In the style of Murrle, Bennett & Co.

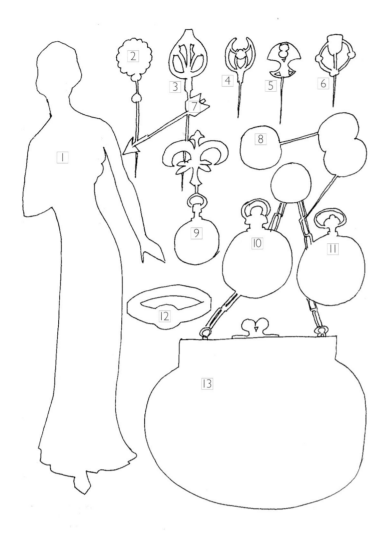

Miscellaneous Jewelry and Jewelled Pieces 1900–1919

1 *c.* 1911. Pierced bandeau of white paste stones, matching pendant earrings, shoulder clasps, fringed dress garniture under bust and on side-hip level; oval shoe-buckles. 2 *c.* 1900. Gold hatpin, large ball head covered in seed pearls. 3 *c.* 1902. Silver hatpin, pierced head, thistle design. In the style of Arabella Rankin. 4 *c.* 1902. Gold scarf pin set with central amethyst. In the style of V. Schönthoner. 5 *c.* 1902. Fan-shaped gold scarf pin set with coloured stones. In the style of Otto Prutscher. 6 *c.* 1902. Gold scarf pin set with turquoise stones. 7 *c.* 1919. Gold arrow hat ornament, set with diamonds, synthetic sapphire trim. 8 *c.* 1919. Two large blown-glass pearl-effect hatpins, metal pins and fixings. 9 *c.* 1912. Enamelled corsage watch, centrally set pearls and diamonds, matching outer edge, foliate brooch set in similar manner. 10 *c.* 1910. Gold watch, plain hunting case with raised two-colour gold monogram. 11 *c.* 1900. Gold pocket watch, case decorated in multicoloured enamels, swirling daisy design. In the style of René Lalique. 12 *c.* 1918. Gold watch bracelet, shoulders set with diamonds in floral design, mother-of-pearl face, diamond surround. 13 *c.* 1918. Silk evening bag, multicoloured glass-bead embroidery design of flowers and leaves, solid single-colour glass-bead background, enamelled silver frame, long linked chain handle, amber bead clasp fastening.

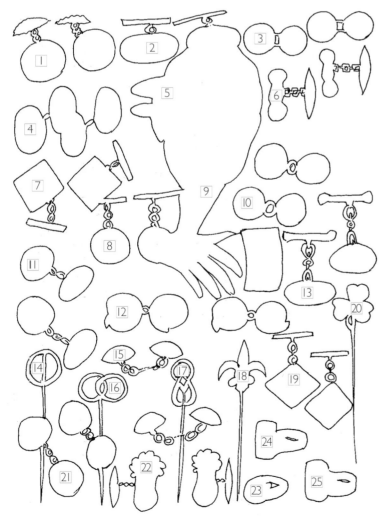

Men's Jewelry 1900–1919

1 *c.* 1900. Gold cufflinks, multicoloured mosaic plaques. 2 *c.* 1900. Gold cufflinks, plaques depicting dogs. 3 *c.* 1910. Silver cufflinks, ivory plaques set with pearl, coloured-enamel surround. 4 *c.* 1903. Gold cufflinks, engraved oval plaques. 5 *c.* 1901. Gold cuff studs, engraved front plaques, plain backs. 6 *c.* 1902. Gold bar cufflinks. 7 *c.* 1904. Gold cufflinks, carved glass plaques. 8 *c.* 1905. Gold cufflinks, round enamelled plaques, four-leaf-clover design. 9 *c.* 1910. Gold stickpin set with synthetic cabochon ruby, gold signet ring, gold cufflinks central pearl, pearl surround. 10 *c.* 1908. Gold cufflinks, circular plaques, set with blue chalcedony, gold and white enamelled key pattern border. In the style of Fabergé. 11 *c.* 1909. Jade cufflinks, set with bars of rubies and diamonds, gold chain connections. In the style of Alexander Tillander. 12 *c.* 1900. Gold cufflinks, serpent surrounding cabochon garnet. 13 *c.* 1915. Gold cufflinks, oval opal plaques, ruby, diamond and sapphire surround, ruby endstones to bar. 14 *c.* 1917. Gold stickpin, open circular head set with rubies. 15 *c.* 1905. Egg-shaped coloured-stone cufflinks banded in diamonds. 16 *c.* 1919. Gold stickpin, head interlocking open circles set with sapphires and diamonds. 17 *c.* 1919. Gold stickpin, head interlocking open pear-shapes set with diamonds and sapphires. 18 *c.* 1900. Gold stickpin, fleur-de-lys head set with pearls. 19 *c.* 1903. Silver cufflinks, carved plaques, set with coloured stone. 20 *c.* 1905. Silver stickpin, enamelled shamrock head. 21 *c.* 1908. Silver cufflinks, button plaques set with coloured stones. 22 *c.* 1906. Silver-gilt cufflinks, wire decoration, set with coloured stones. 23 *c.* 1905. Gold ring set with cabochon stone, carved shoulders. 24 *c.* 1900. Gold ring, rectangular onyx stone, diamond set initial, open shoulders. 25 *c.* 1908. Gold ring, large coloured stone.

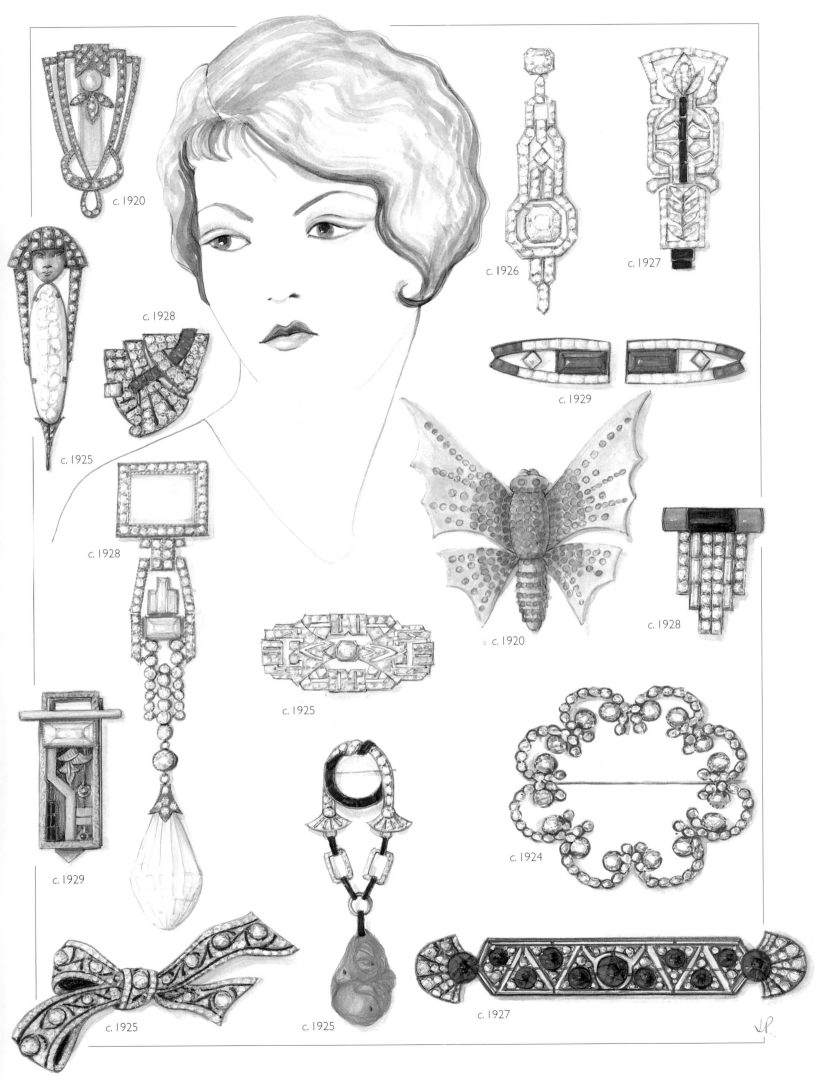

c. 1920

c. 1928

c. 1925

c. 1928

c. 1926

c. 1927

c. 1929

c. 1920

c. 1928

c. 1925

c. 1929

c. 1924

c. 1925

c. 1925

c. 1927

Earrings 1920–1929

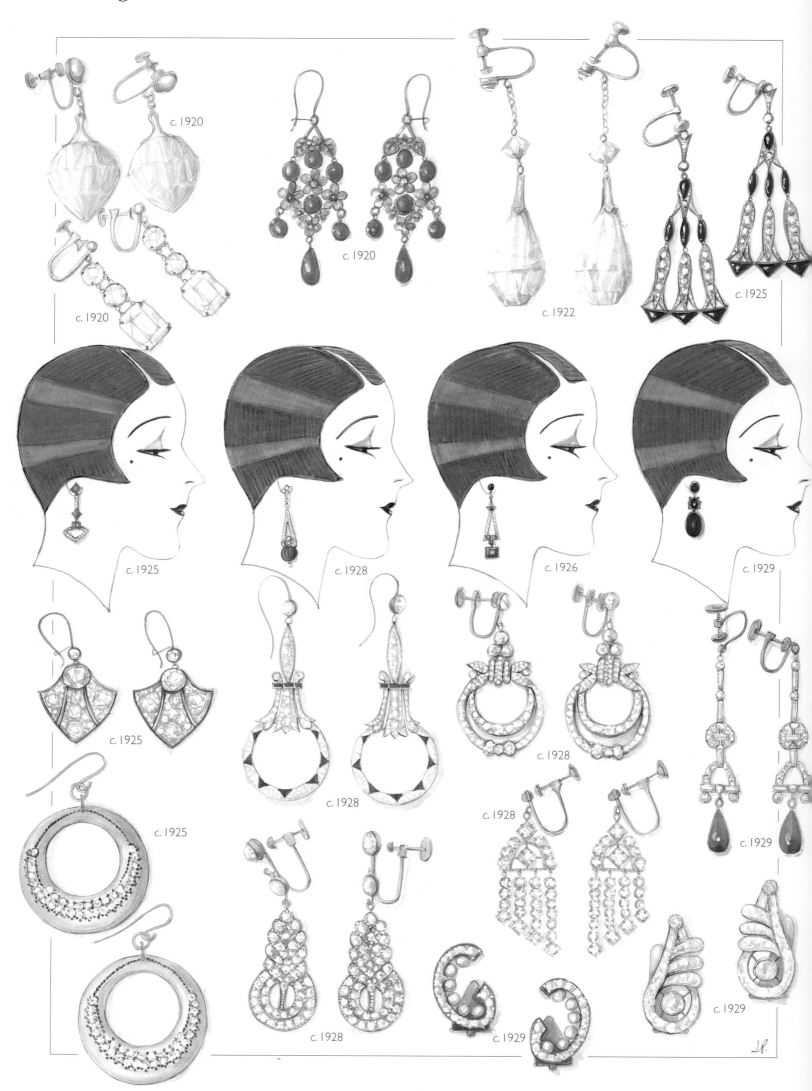

c. 1920

c. 1920

c. 1920

c. 1922

c. 1925

c. 1925

c. 1928

c. 1926

c. 1929

c. 1925

c. 1928

c. 1928

c. 1929

c. 1925

c. 1928

c. 1928

c. 1929

c. 1929

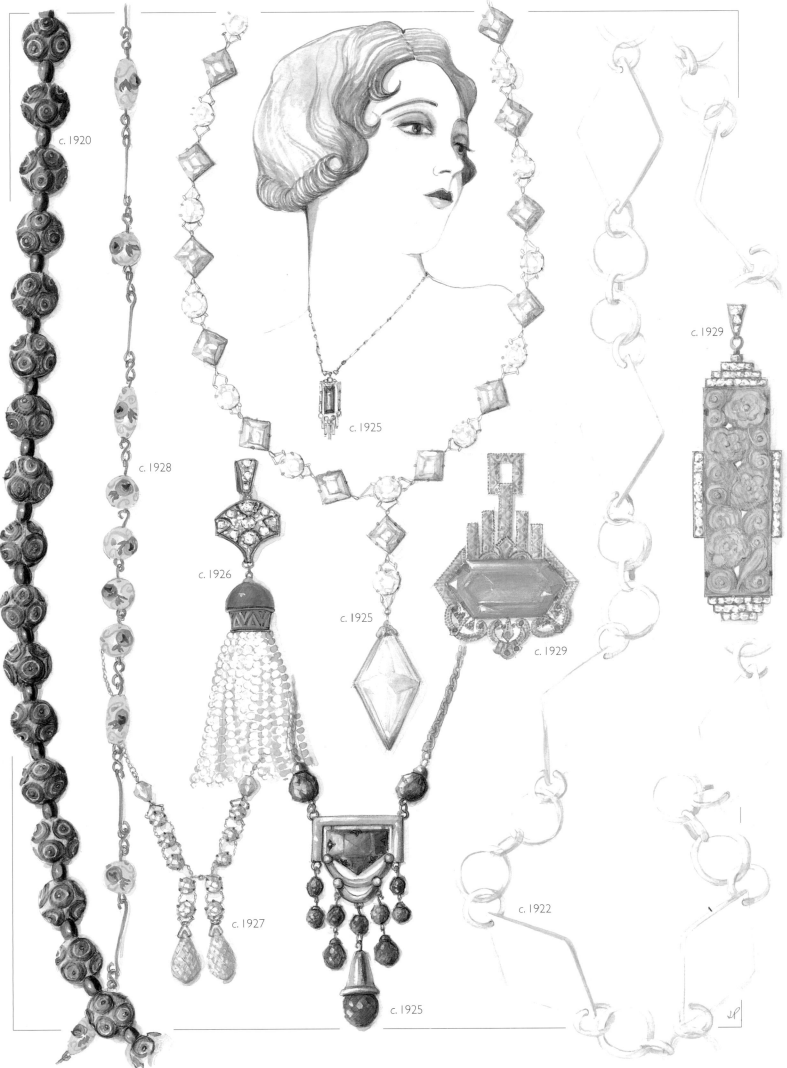

c. 1920

c. 1928

c. 1926

c. 1927

c. 1925

c. 1925

c. 1925

c. 1929

c. 1929

c. 1922

c. 1925

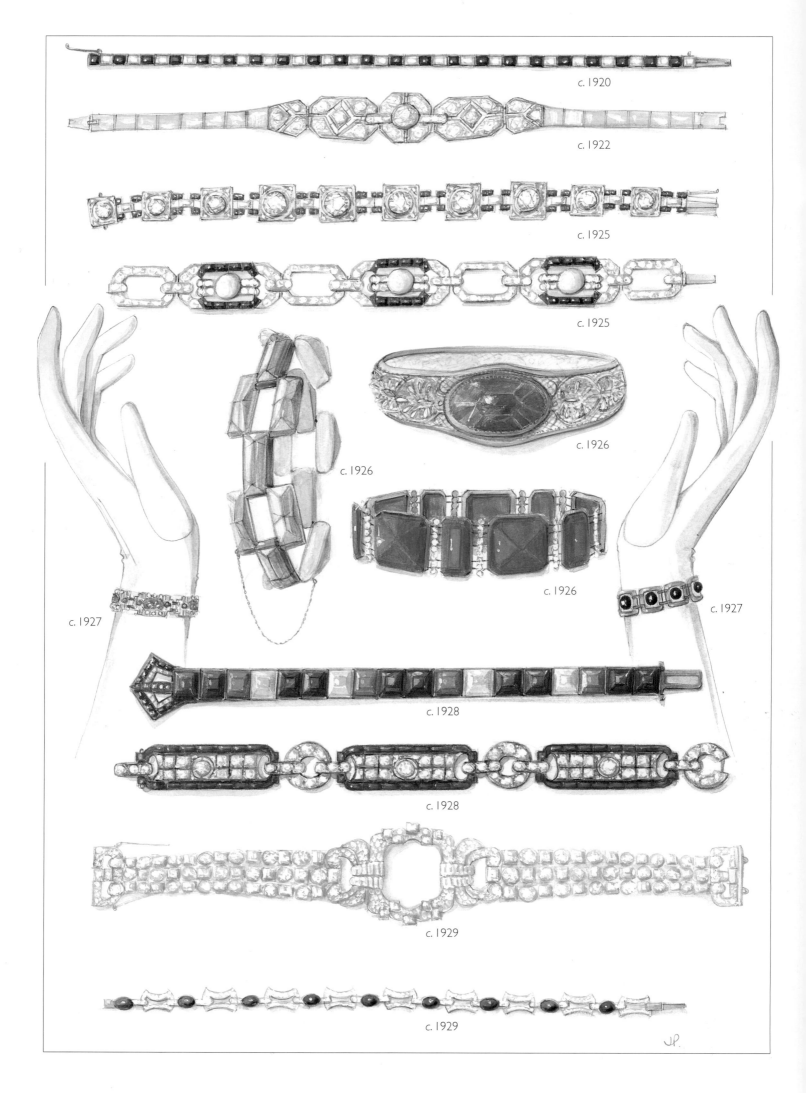

c. 1920

c. 1922

c. 1925

c. 1925

c. 1926

c. 1926

c. 1926

c. 1927

c. 1927

c. 1928

c. 1928

c. 1929

c. 1929

JP.

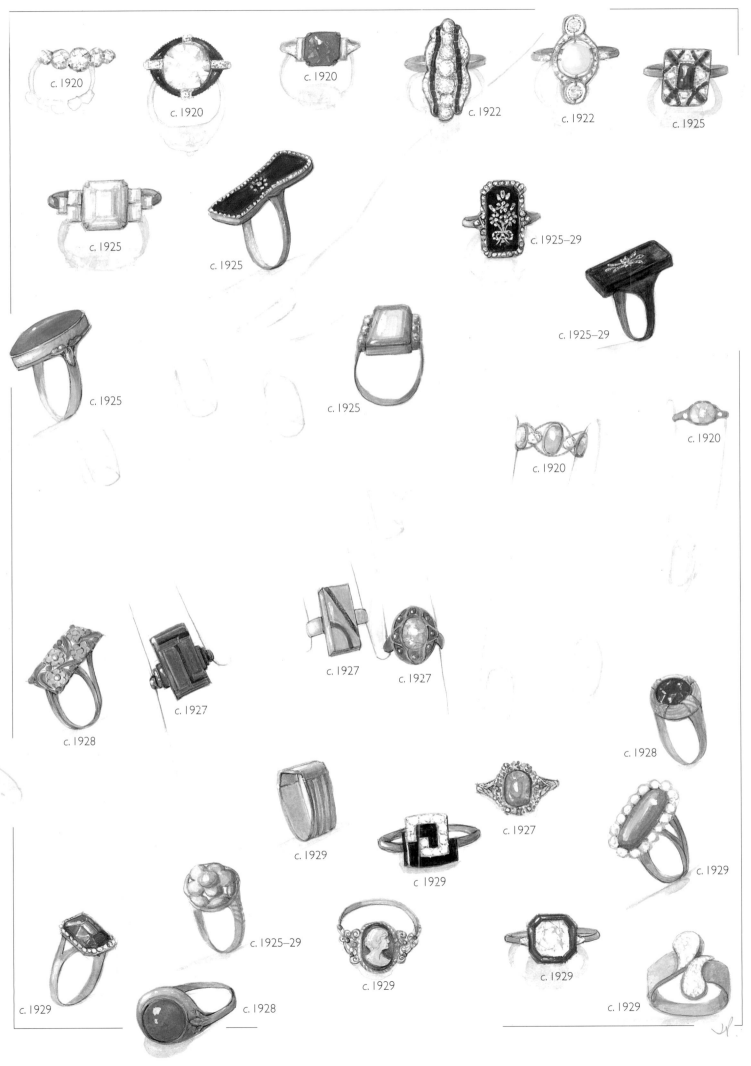

c. 1920

c. 1920

c. 1920

c. 1922

c. 1922

c. 1925

c. 1925

c. 1925

c. 1925–29

c. 1925–29

c. 1925

c. 1925

c. 1920

c. 1920

c. 1928

c. 1927

c. 1927

c. 1927

c. 1928

c. 1929

c. 1929

c. 1927

c. 1929

c. 1929

c. 1925–29

c. 1929

c. 1928

c. 1929

c. 1929

c. 1929

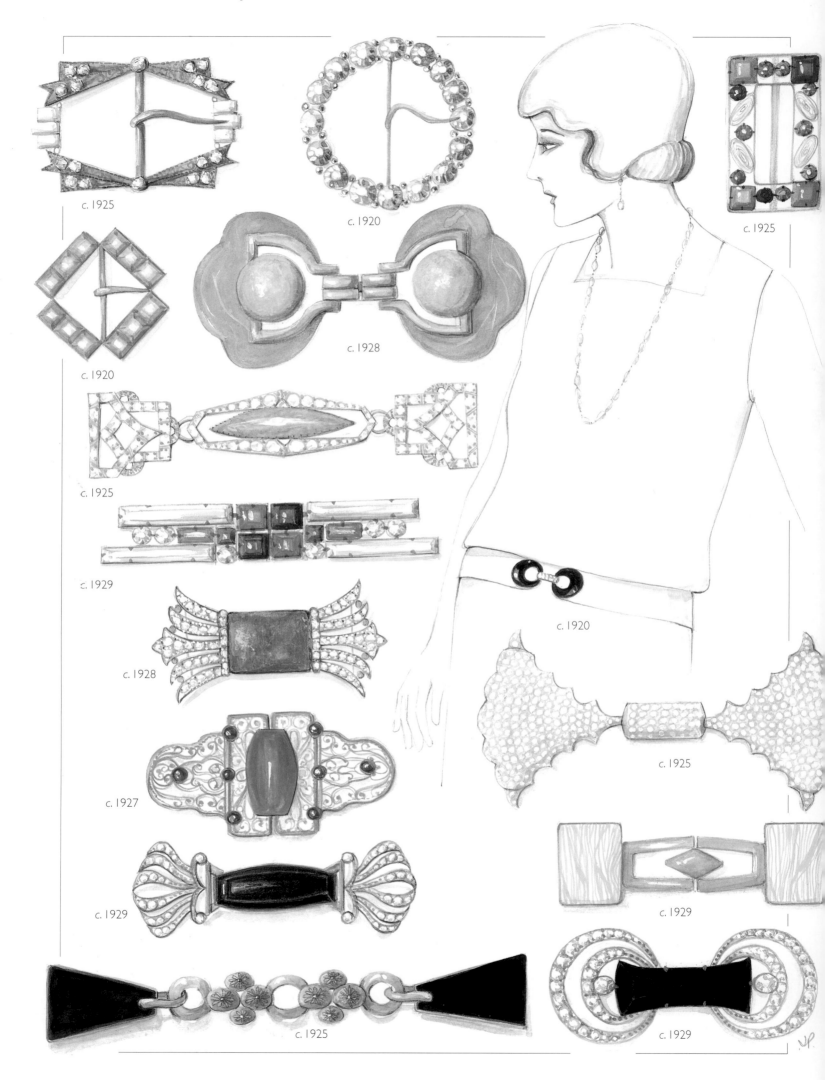

c. 1925

c. 1920

c. 1925

c. 1920

c. 1928

c. 1925

c. 1929

c. 1920

c. 1928

c. 1925

c. 1927

c. 1929

c. 1929

c. 1925

c. 1929

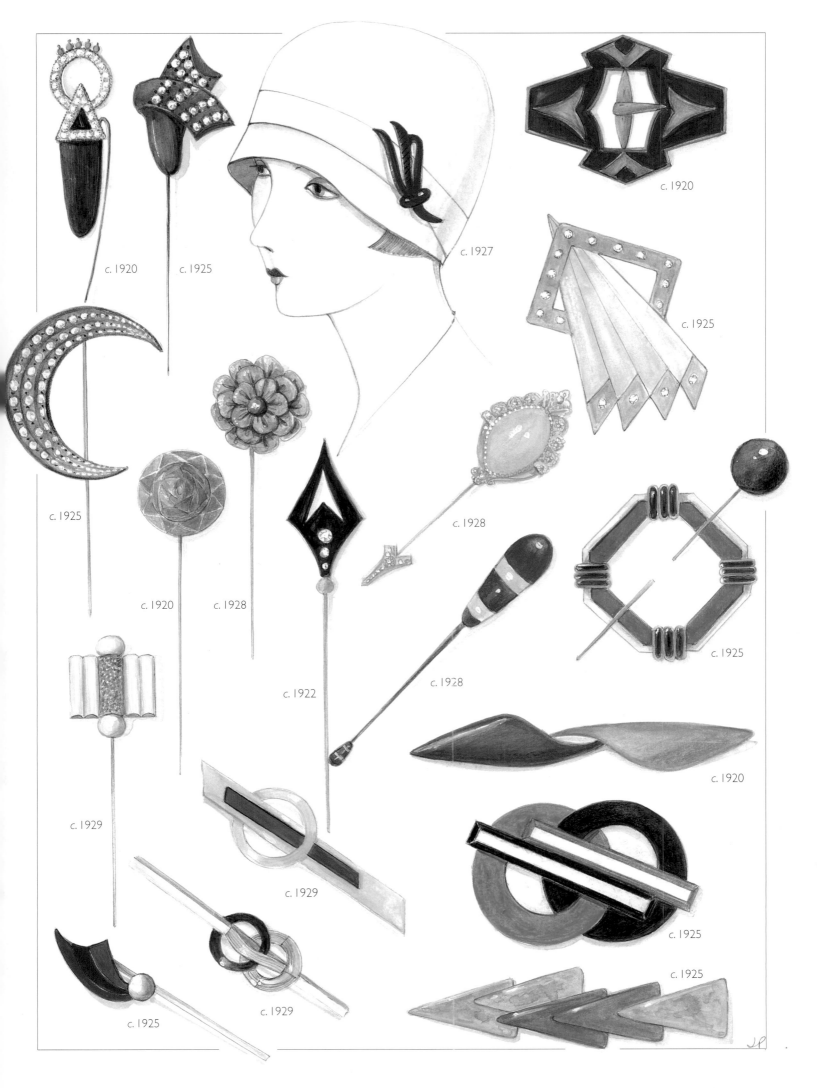

c. 1920

c. 1925

c. 1927

c. 1920

c. 1925

c. 1925

c. 1925

c. 1920

c. 1928

c. 1928

c. 1922

c. 1928

c. 1925

c. 1929

c. 1920

c. 1929

c. 1925

c. 1925

c. 1925

c. 1929

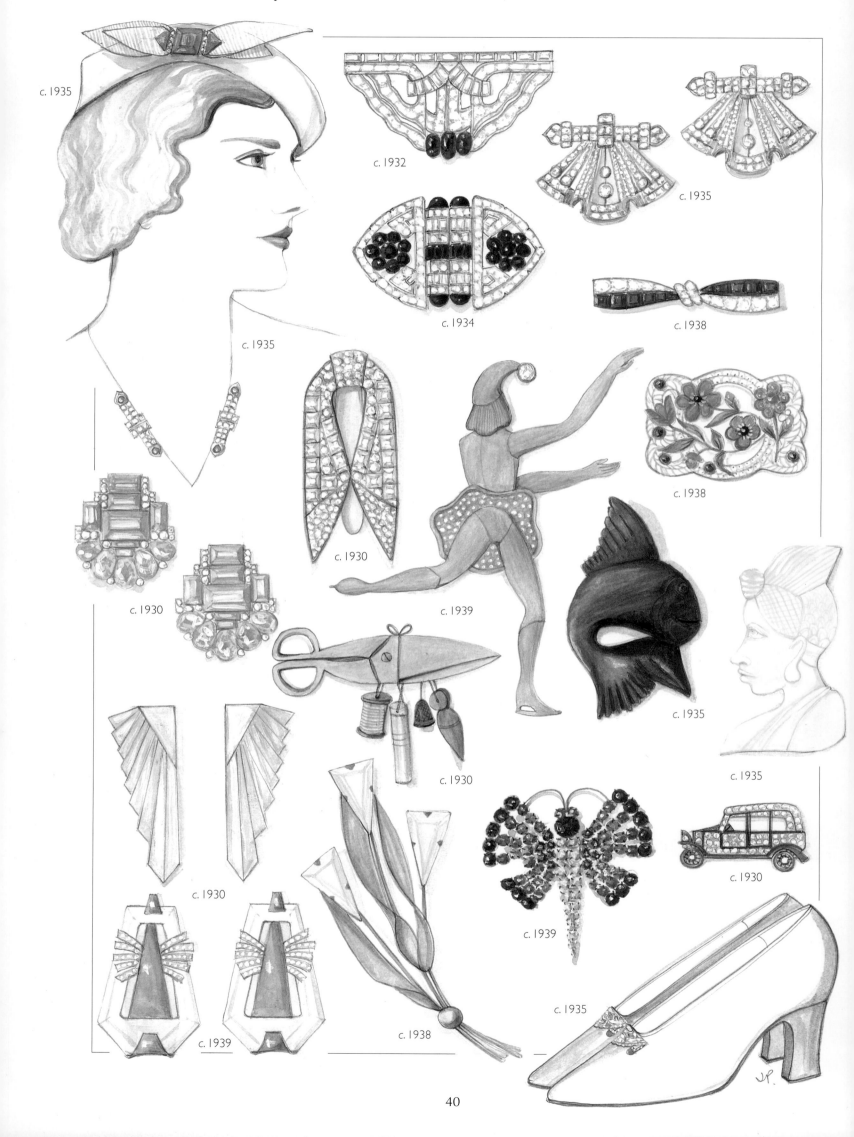

c. 1935

c. 1932

c. 1935

c. 1934

c. 1938

c. 1935

c. 1938

c. 1930

c. 1930

c. 1930

c. 1939

c. 1935

c. 1935

c. 1930

c. 1930

c. 1930

c. 1939

c. 1938

c. 1939

c. 1930

c. 1935

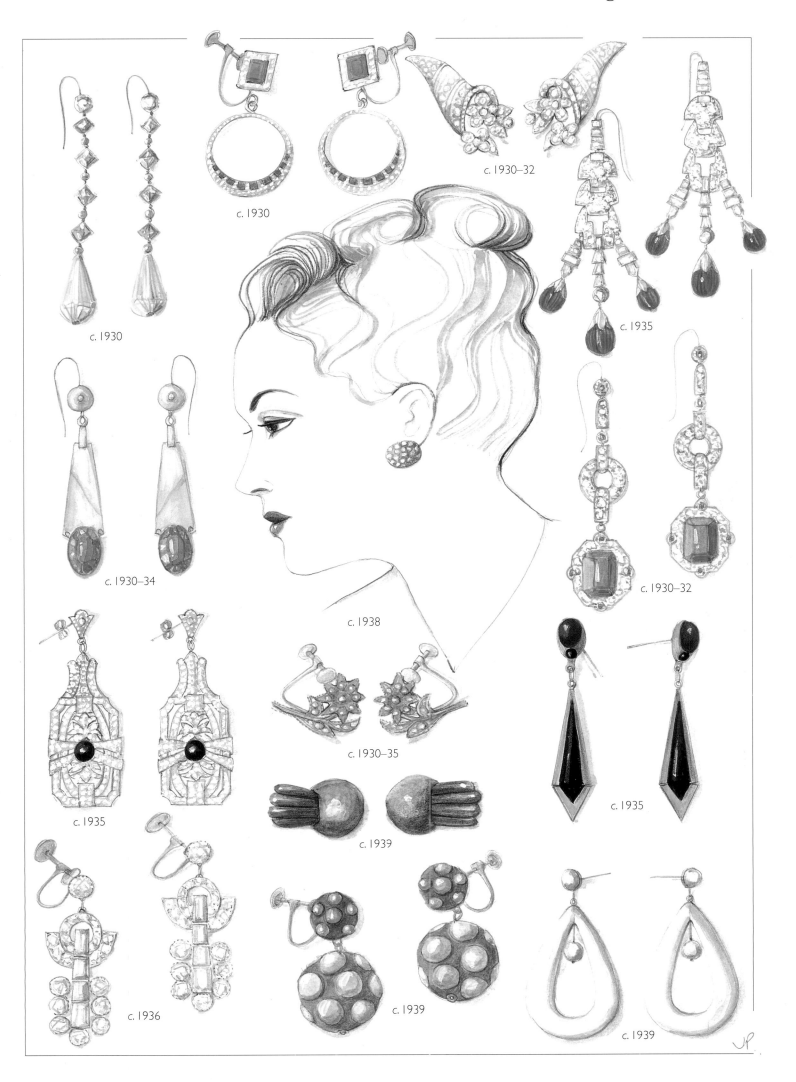

c. 1930–32

c. 1930

c. 1930

c. 1935

c. 1930–34

c. 1930–32

c. 1938

c. 1935

c. 1930–35

c. 1935

c. 1939

c. 1936

c. 1939

c. 1939

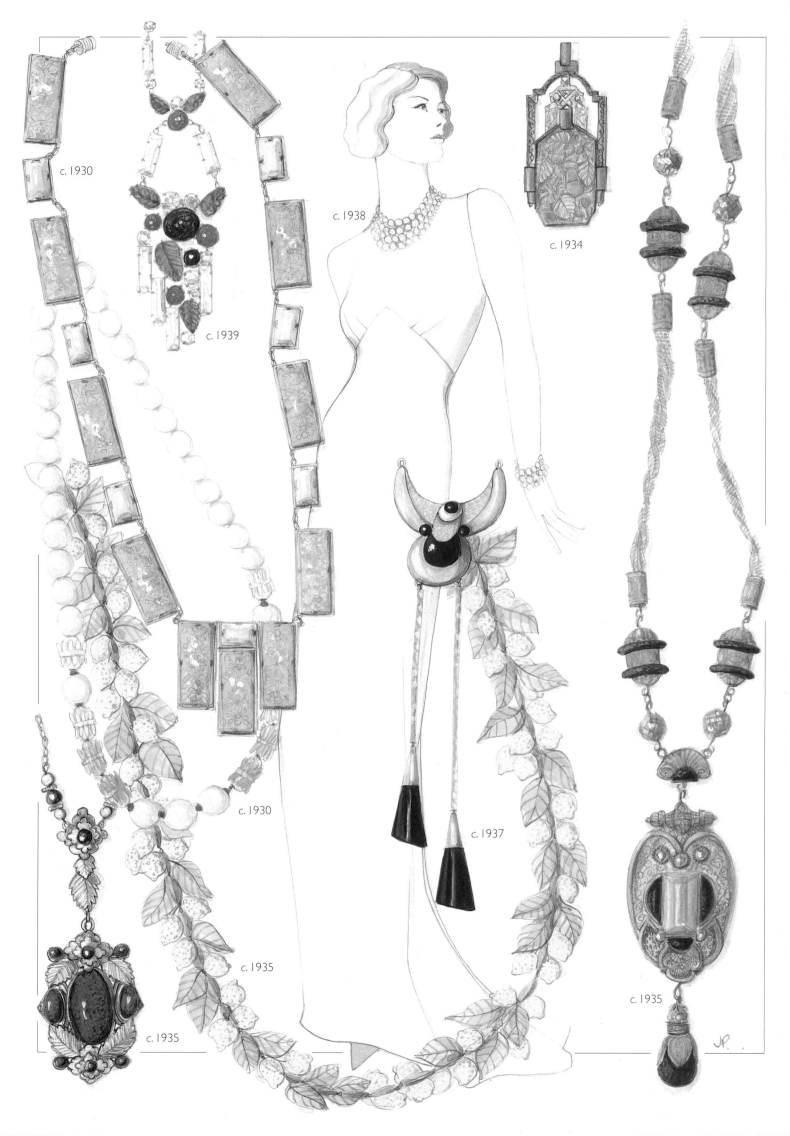

c. 1930

c. 1939

c. 1938

c. 1934

c. 1930

c. 1937

c. 1935

c. 1935

c. 1935

JP.

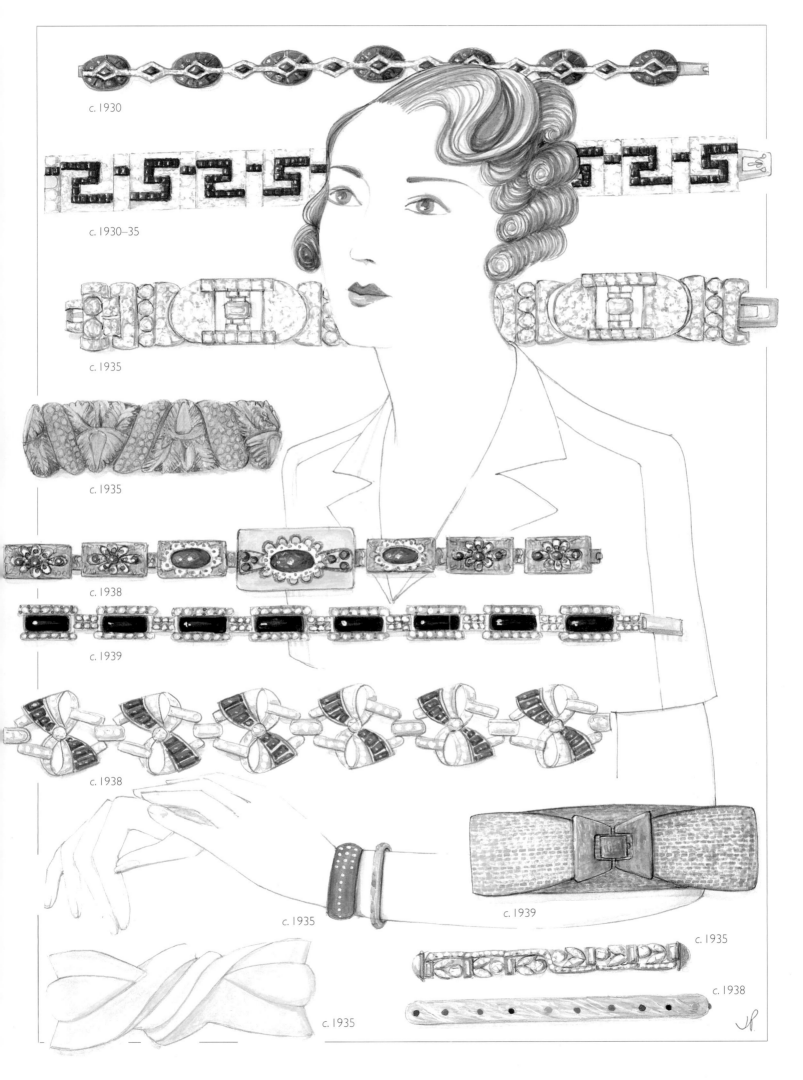

c.1930

c.1930–35

c.1935

c.1935

c.1938

c.1939

c.1938

c.1935

c.1939

c.1935

c.1935

c.1938

Rings 1930–1939

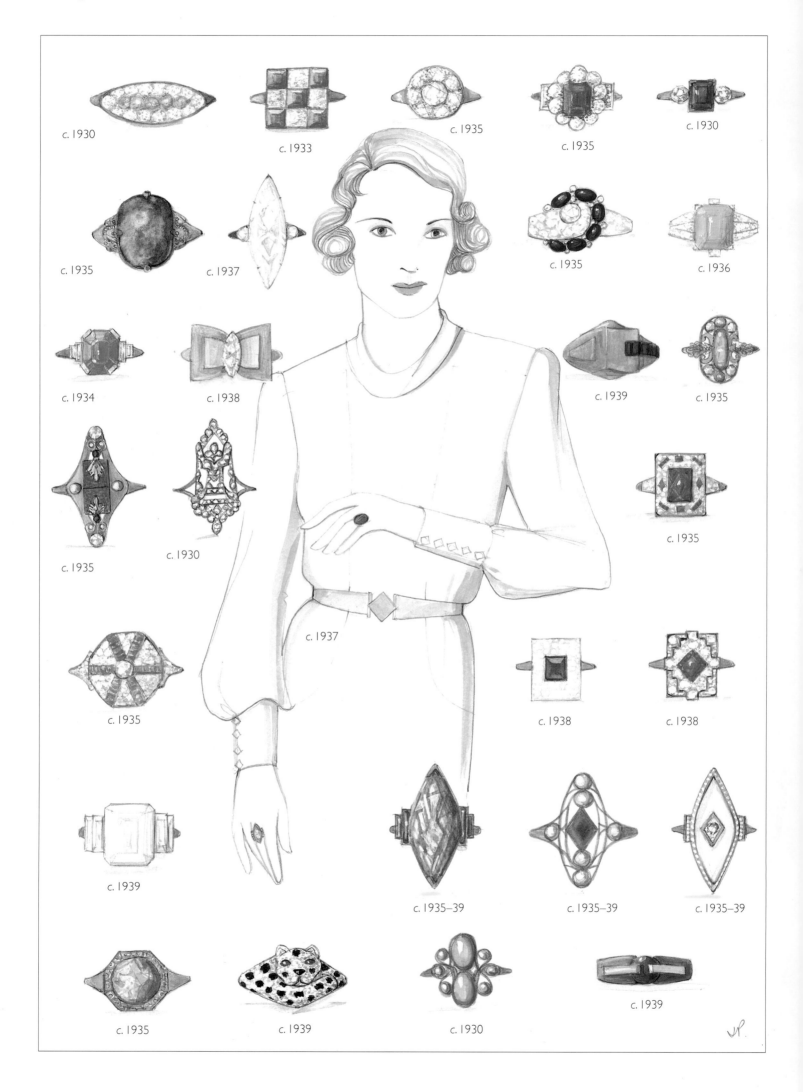

c. 1930

c. 1933

c. 1935

c. 1935

c. 1930

c. 1935

c. 1937

c. 1935

c. 1936

c. 1934

c. 1938

c. 1939

c. 1935

c. 1935

c. 1930

c. 1935

c. 1937

c. 1935

c. 1938

c. 1938

c. 1939

c. 1935–39

c. 1935–39

c. 1935–39

c. 1935

c. 1939

c. 1930

c. 1939

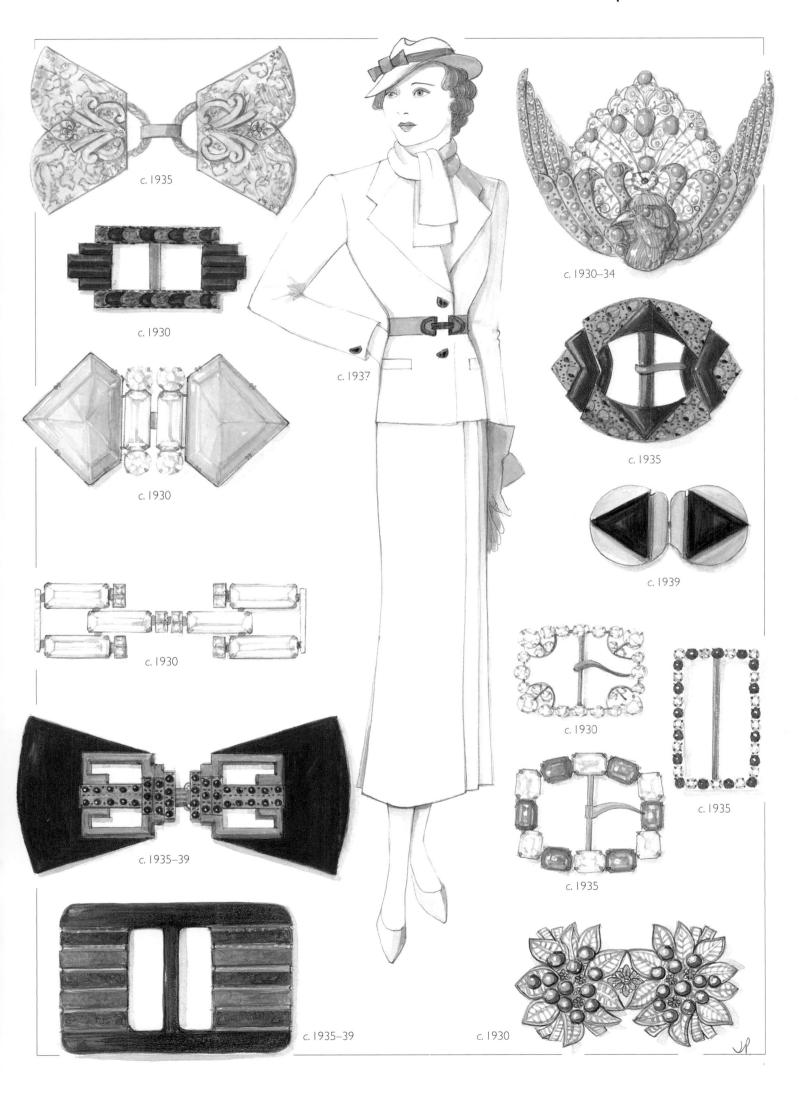

c. 1935

c. 1930

c. 1930

c. 1930

c. 1935–39

c. 1935–39

c. 1937

c. 1930–34

c. 1935

c. 1939

c. 1930

c. 1935

c. 1935

c. 1930

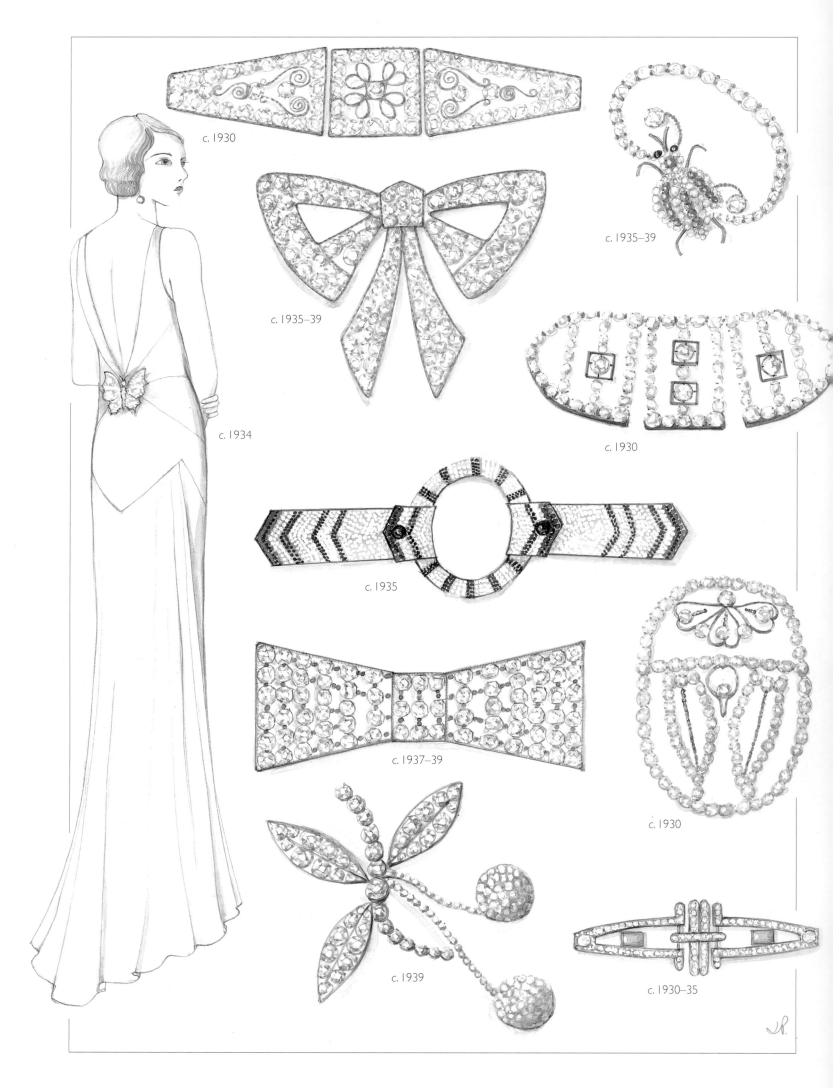

c.1930

c.1935–39

c.1935–39

c.1934

c.1930

c.1935

c.1930

c.1937–39

c.1930

c.1939

c.1930–35

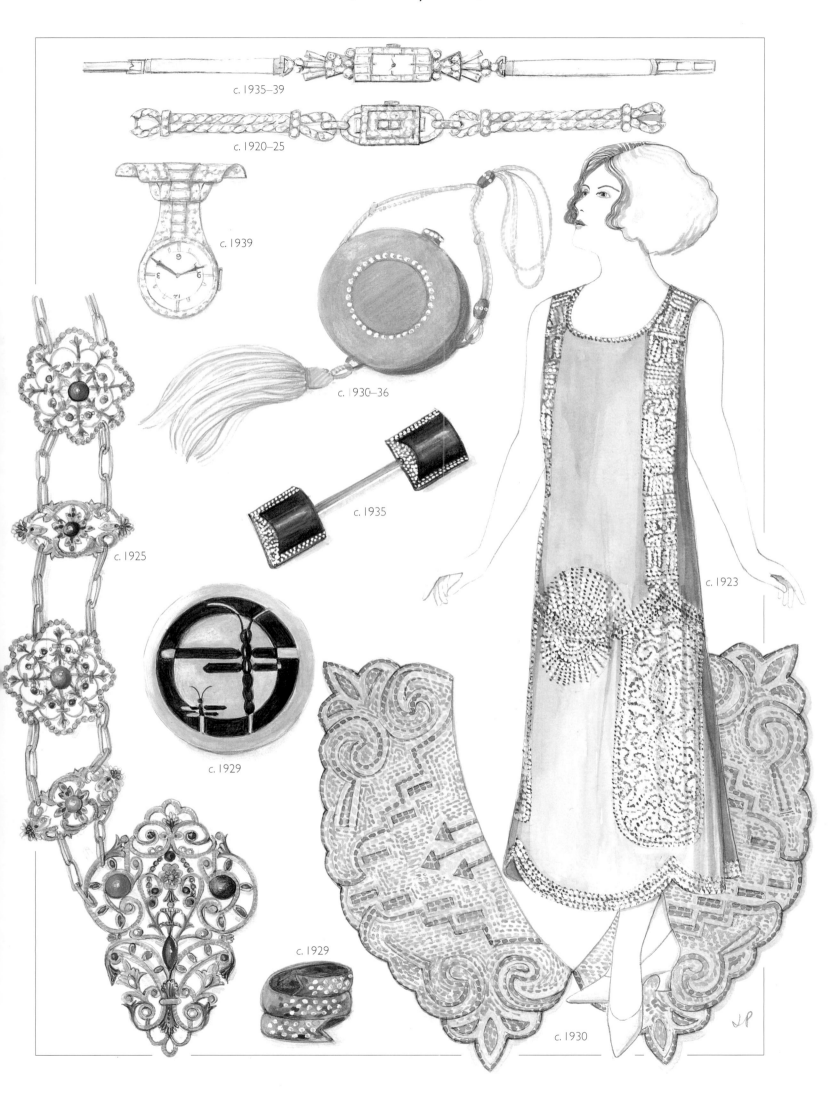

c. 1935–39

c. 1920–25

c. 1939

c. 1930–36

c. 1935

c. 1925

c. 1929

c. 1923

c. 1929

c. 1930

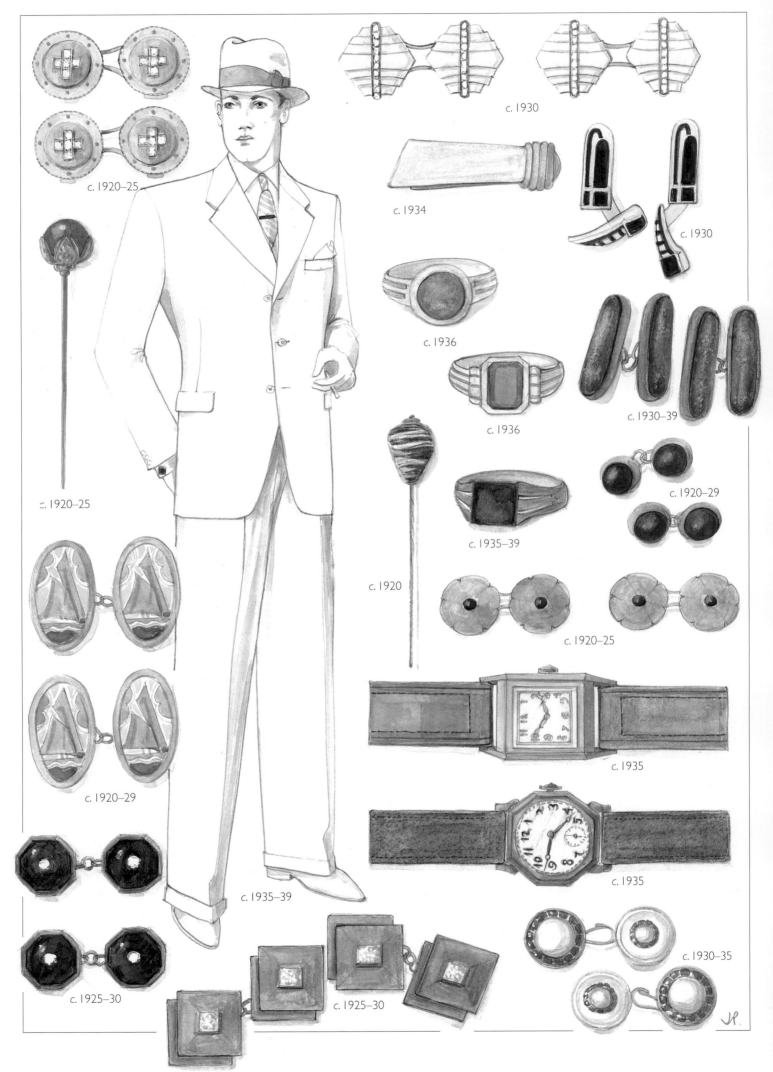

c. 1920–25

c. 1930

c. 1930

c. 1934

c. 1930

c. 1936

c. 1920–25

c. 1936

c. 1930–39

c. 1920–29

c. 1920–29

c. 1935–39

c. 1920

c. 1920–25

c. 1935

c. 1935–39

c. 1935

c. 1930–35

c. 1925–30

c. 1925–30

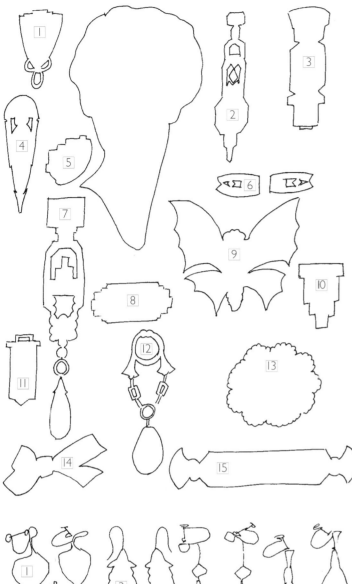

Brooches and Clips 1920–1929

1 *c.* 1920. Pierced shield-shaped silver dress clip, set with marcasites, single centrally placed fake pearl. 2 *c.* 1926. Geometric platinum brooch, set with brilliant-cut diamonds, diamond-set borders.
3 *c.* 1927. Pierced-silver dress clip, set with white paste stones, line of fake rubies, matching base. 4 *c.* 1925. Egyptian-revival-style metal brooch, set with marcasites, engraved oval plastic panel under carved portrait. 5 *c.* 1928. Diamond and sapphire clasp, scroll design.
6 *c.* 1929. Pair of metal dress clips, set with fake emeralds and diamonds. 7 *c.* 1928. Silver pendant brooch, rectangular clear paste stone, marcasite surround, matching hinged pendant supporting large clear paste peardrop. 8 *c.* 1925. Diamond-set plaque brooch, pierced mount. 9 *c.* 1920. Cream plastic moth brooch, carved body and outstretched scalloped wings decorated with tiny sequins. 10 *c.* 1928. Metal clasp, fake onyx and amber bar supporting graded lines of white paste stones. 11 *c.* 1929. Metal clasp, pierced oriental design, small panel of painted enamel, large white paste stone under hinge.
12 *c.* 1925. Pendant brooch, ruby and diamond set with twisted ribbon hoop and tassels matching bars and rectangular links supporting carved jade drop. 13 *c.* 1924. Brooch of white paste stones set into scalloped metal frame. 14 *c.* 1925. Tied bow knot, waved ends, set with lines of graded brilliant-cut diamonds, diamond-set background, pierced lines to accentuate design. 15 *c.* 1927. Novelty bar brooch, Christmas-cracker design, set with sapphires and diamonds, pierced chevron decoration.

Earrings 1920–1929

1 *c.* 1920. Transparent blue glass pendant earrings, metal fixings, screw fasteners. 2 *c.* 1920. Transparent moulded-glass pendant earrings, metal fixings, screw fasteners. 3 *c.* 1920. Gilded-brass earrings, floral design, set with simulated turquoise stones. 4 *c.* 1922. Transparent pink glass pendant earrings, large moulded pear-shaped drops suspended below matching bead, silver fixings, screw fasteners.
5 *c.* 1925. Silver-gilt pendant earrings, three joined droplets set with synthetic rubies and diamonds. 6 *c.* 1925. Pendant earrings, set with coloured glass and marcasites. 7 *c.* 1928. Pendant earrings set with marcasites, ribbed synthetic sapphire ball. 8 *c.* 1926. Silver pendant earrings, set with square amethysts. 9 *c.* 1929. Metal pendant earrings, set with coloured-plastic stones. 10 *c.* 1925. Pierced shield-shaped earrings, set with old-cut diamonds, matching surmount. 11 *c.* 1928. Pendant earrings, open hoops set with triangular-cut synthetic sapphires, diamond surround, matching scroll-design top. 12 *c.* 1928. Pendant earrings, double open hoops, set with white paste stones, matching foliate and surmount. 13 *c.* 1929. Long pendant earrings, set with clear paste stones, uncut synthetic emerald teardrops. 14 *c.* 1925. Coloured-plastic hoop earrings, set with rows of marcasites and tiny gold-coloured metal studs. 15 *c.* 1928. Metal pendant earrings, foliate design above open hoop, set with marcasites. 16 *c.* 1929. C-shaped gold clip earrings, set with diamonds, inner border of cultured pearls.
17 *c.* 1928. Asymmetric pendant earrings, set with white paste stones.
18 *c.* 1929. Platinum clip earrings, scroll design set with diamonds.

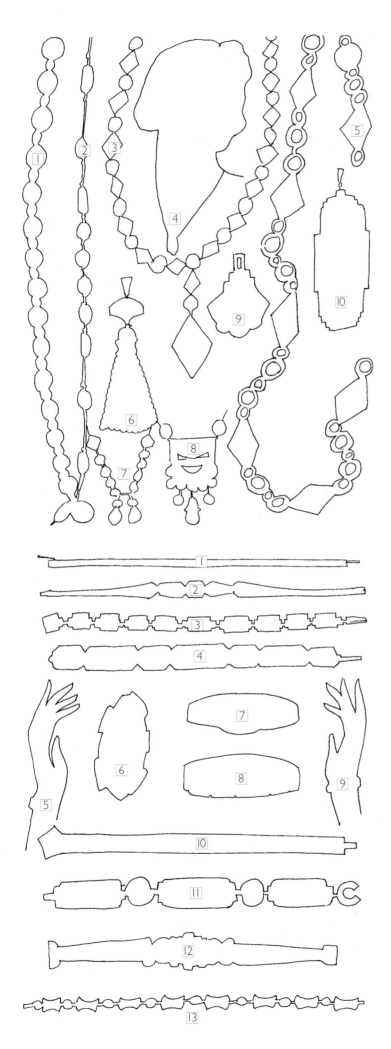

Necklaces and Pendants 1920–1929

1 *c.* 1920. Long necklace of carved and painted round wooden beads, spaced by small painted oval wooden beads. 2 *c.* 1928. Long opaque turquoise-coloured glass-bead necklace, raised multicoloured flower and leaf decoration, spaced by single beads and flat gold-coloured metal-wire linking rods. 3 *c.* 1925. Transparent two-colour glass-bead necklace, matching large diamond-shaped pendant, fine silver wire links and fixings. 4 *c.* 1925. Oblong transparent blue glass pendant within a frame of clear glass stones, suspended from a glass stone and silver wire chain. 5 *c.* 1922. Long plastic-ivory necklace, diamond-shaped plates, connected by sets of rings in matching plastic. 6 *c.* 1926. Platinum pendant with shield-shaped surmount set with diamonds, supporting half a jade bead set into engraved band above seed-pearl tassel. In the style of Tiffany & Co. 7 *c.* 1927. Moulded coloured flat glass-bead necklace ending in two teardrops, silver fixings and fine chain back. 8 *c.* 1925. Moulded coloured glass-bead necklace, large flat stone set within pewter frame, bead drops, central teardrop with pewter cap, flat chain back. 9 *c.* 1929. Large engraved-metal pendant, angular design, pierced scroll base, large asymmetric moulded transparent fake aquamarine as central setting. 10 *c.* 1929. Carved plastic-jade pendant, pierced floral design, oblong plate banded in metal on four sides set with paste stones, matching support link.

Bracelets 1920–1929

1 *c.* 1920. Narrow gold bracelet, set alternately with square rubies and diamonds. In the style of Cartier. 2 *c.* 1922. Bracelet centrally set with cushion-cut diamond, diamond frame, linking bars to similarly set side bars, polished section back. 3 *c.* 1925. Bracelet composed of ten graduated square plaques each set with brilliant-cut diamond within diamond frame, connected by calibré-cut sapphire and diamond brick links. 4 *c.* 1925. Bracelet composed of three oblong open plaques centrally set with faux pearl, synthetic diamond and onyx surround, connected by openwork plaques. 5 *c.* 1927. Bracelet of oblong polished-metal plates, set with carved plastic central panels, matching stones at each side, hinged links. 6 *c.* 1926. Two-colour gold bracelet, faceted brick-link design, fine catch and safety chain. 7 *c.* 1926. Gold-coloured bracelet, openwork design of palm trees, large centrally set moulded green glass stone. 8 *c.* 1926. Linked bracelet, square moulded coloured-glass plaques set in aluminium frames, matching alternate narrow plaques, spaced by rods set with paste stones. 9 *c.* 1927. Polished-brass bracelet, square plaques set with fake cabochon rubies, chain links. 10 *c.* 1928. Belt-and-buckle bracelet, set with three-colour cushion-shaped moulded-glass stones. 11 *c.* 1928. Bracelet of three oblong articulated panels edged with sapphires, centrally set diamonds, hoop and bar diamond-set connections. 12 *c.* 1929. Bracelet, open buckle-shaped central panel set with diamonds, flexible tapered line of square and round diamonds. 13 *c.* 1929. Narrow bracelet, small open panels set with diamonds, matching connections spaced by cabochon sapphires.

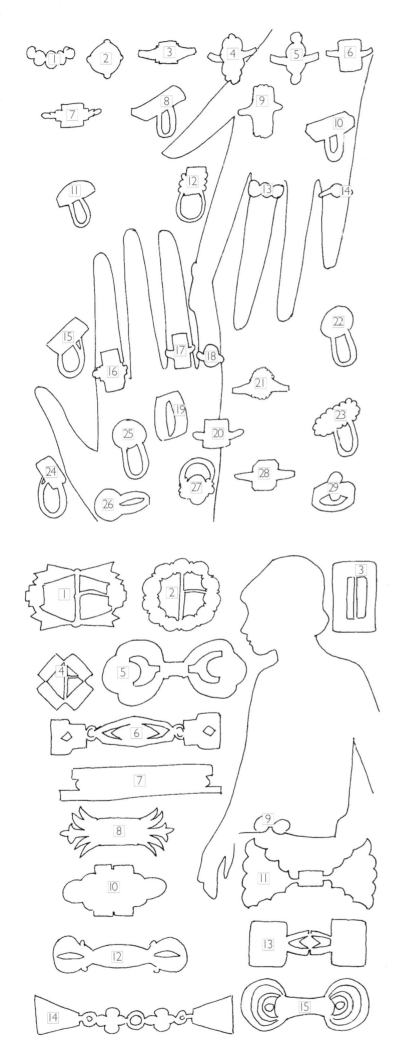

Rings 1920–1929

1 c. 1920. Five-stone claw-set diamond ring, graduated stones.
2 c. 1920. Cushion-cut diamond ring, raised calibré-cut synthetic-sapphire and diamond surround. 3 c. 1920. Cushion-shaped sapphire ring, diamond shoulders. 4 c. 1922. Vertical line of old-cut diamonds, undulating border of sapphires and diamonds. 5 c. 1922. Cultured-pearl ring, diamonds set vertically in oval frame. 6 c. 1925. Cushion-shaped sapphire, matching radiating lines, diamond background.
7 c. 1925. Cushion-shaped glass stone, matching shoulders.
8 c. 1925. Shaped flat stone, seed-pearl centre, matching border.
9 c. 1925–29. Oblong plaque, marcasite design. 10 c. 1925–29. Black Bakelite ring, rhinestone setting. 11 c. 1925. Polished-glass stone set in silver, decorative shoulders. 12 c. 1925. Oblong coloured-glass stone, matching shoulders. 13 c. 1920. Graduated opals and diamonds, gold wire frame. 14 c. 1920. Round coloured-glass stone, fake-pearl shoulders. 15 c. 1928. Pierced enamelled ring, flower design, split shoulders. 16 c. 1927. Rectangular ring, abstract design, multicoloured enamels, step shoulders. 17 c. 1927. Rectangular plaque, enamelled abstract design. 18 c. 1927. Round smoky quartz ring, gold wire surround set with small turquoise stones. 19 c. 1929. Gold band, lapis lines. In the style of Jean Fouquet. 20 c. 1929. Enamel and diamond ring, Greek key pattern. In the style of Raymond Templier. 21 c. 1927. Cushion-shaped coloured-glass stone, silver bead surround. 22 c. 1928. Ruby set in engraved-gold mount. 23 c. 1929. Oval emerald, pearl surround. 24 c. 1929. Cushion-shaped coloured-glass ring, seed-pearl surround. 25 c. 1925–29. Carved and moulded coloured-glass ring.
26 c. 1928. Jadite stone, decorative shoulders. 27 c. 1929. Cameo set in silver, scroll shoulders. 28 c. 1929. Diamond set in hexagonal synthetic-sapphire mount. 29 c. 1929. Split-gold band, diamond trim. In the style of Raymond Templier.

Buckles and Clasps 1920–1929

1 c. 1925. Polished-brass dress buckle, ribbed-wire decoration, set with rhinestones, clear glass baguettes at each side panel, single prong.
2 c. 1920. Round brass dress buckle, set with coloured-glass stones spaced by small rhinestones, single prong. 3 c. 1925. Oblong gold-coloured metal belt-buckle, set with multicoloured stones and decorated with ribbed wire. 4 c. 1920. Polished-brass buckle, square bezel set with amber-coloured stones, single prong. 5 c. 1928. Green plastic marble-look dress clasp, decorated with gold painted balls, matching other trim and fastening. 6 c. 1925. Long pierced-silver belt clasp, central pointed oval opal stone, surround and end clips set with rhinestones. 7 c. 1929. Belt clasp of graded rectangular transparent-coloured moulded-glass stones, set off by six small clear moulded-glass stones, central clip fastening. 8 c. 1928. Silver clasp, central rectangular stone, leaf-shaped side spray panels set with rhinestones. 9 c. 1920. Pressed-glass belt clasp of two pierced discs joined by pavé-set paste stone bar. 10 c. 1927. Openwork gold-coloured wire belt clasp, set with coloured-glass stones, oblong central coloured-plastic stone covering fastening. 11 c. 1925. Bow-shaped metal belt clasp, scalloped edges set with rhinestones, matching cylindrical central bar, side screw fastening.
12 c. 1929. Silver-gilt clasp, oblong pressed-glass stone, scroll-design sides set with rhinestones. 13 c. 1929. Polished-aluminium belt clasp, central fastening, rectangular striped-glass side plaques. 14 c. 1925. Clasp comprising textured metal beads and ring connections between triangular black plastic plaques. 15 c. 1929. Prong-set fake-jet clasp, hoop sides set with paste stones.

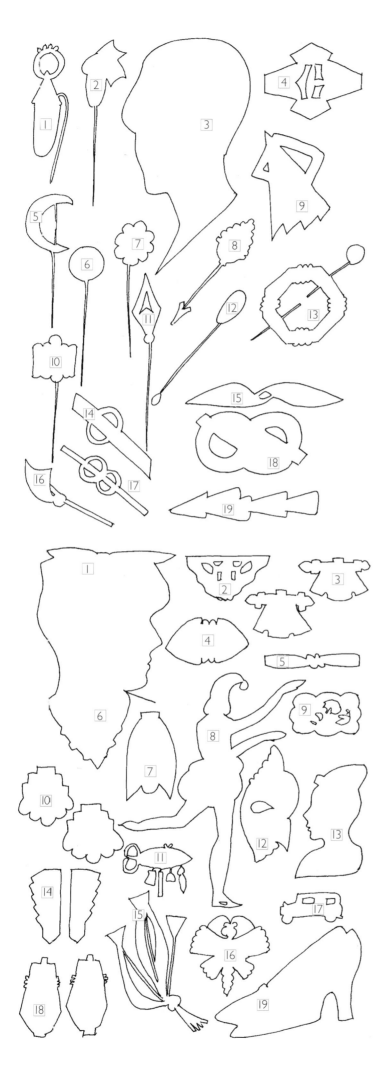

Hat Ornaments 1920–1929

1 *c.* 1920. Plastic shield-shaped hatpin, open triangle and hoop top set with rhinestones, topped with gold beads, curved pin. 2 *c.* 1925. Plastic hatpin, wrapover design, rhinestone trim. 3 *c.* 1927. Red carved-plastic hat ornament, foliate design. 4 *c.* 1920. Gilded-metal fancy-shaped hat-buckle, painted enamel background. 5 *c.* 1925. Crescent-shaped plastic hatpin, set with lines of graduated paste stones and metal beads. 6 *c.* 1920. Two-colour carved-plastic hatpin, central rose motif. 7 *c.* 1928. Suede flower hatpin, glass-bead centre. 8 *c.* 1928. Coloured-glass stone hatpin, moulded base-metal surround, matching endstop. 9 *c.* 1925. Two-colour carved-plastic hat ornament, set with rhinestones, scarf and buckle design. 10 *c.* 1929. Plastic hatpin, speckled cylindrical centrepiece, plastic-bead trim to top and bottom, flanked by similar plain plastic reeds. 11 *c.* 1922. Base-metal spear-shaped hatpin, pierced and painted head, set with paste stones. 12 *c.* 1928. Multicoloured striped glass hatpin, matching endstop. 13 *c.* 1925. Hat fastening in white metal, enamelled blue and black, pin with onyx bead head. In the style of Paul Piel et Fils. 14 *c.* 1929. Chrome hat brooch, matching threaded hoop, coloured-plastic bar trim. 15 *c.* 1920. Two-colour plastic twisted hat ornament. 16 *c.* 1925. Polished base-metal hat brooch, matching ball under painted flag-shaped decoration. 17 *c.* 1929. Chrome hat brooch, matching engraved threaded hoop, second hoop in black plastic. 18 *c.* 1925. Three-colour plastic hat ornament, composed of interlocking hoops and cross bars. 19 *c.* 1925. Hat ornament comprising row of triangular polished-glass stones.

Brooches and Clips 1930–1939

1 *c.* 1935. Moulded coloured-glass hat brooch, square and triangular panels spaced by bars set with white paste stones. 2 *c.* 1932. Brooch set with brilliant- and baguette-cut diamonds in a pierced scroll design, oval sapphires to base. 3 *c.* 1935. Pair of silver-gilt dress clips, fan-shaped motif under bar set with white paste stones. 4 *c.* 1934. Double-clip brooch, plaques set with circular-cut ruby cluster, openwork diamond border, two vertical batons set with baguette-cut diamonds and rubies, cabochon ruby terminals. 5 *c.* 1938. Bow brooch, composed of two lines of brilliant-cut diamonds and synthetic calibré-cut rubies. 6 *c.* 1935. Pair of platinum dress clips, set with brilliant-cut diamonds, shaped terminals set with synthetic cabochon emeralds. 7 *c.* 1930. Gilded-metal dress clip, insect-wing design, set with lines of rectangular white paste stones and small rhinestones. 8 *c.* 1939. Gilded-metal ice-skater brooch, skirt and hat set with white paste stones. 9 *c.* 1938. Gold painted wire brooch, decorated with painted flowers and coloured-glass stones. 10 *c.* 1930. Rectangular and oval aquamarine dress clips within diamond framework. 11 *c.* 1930. Bakelite novelty brooch, scissors and sewing equipment. 12 *c.* 1935. Bakelite novelty brooch, fish design. 13 *c.* 1935. Carved ivory-coloured plastic lapel brooch. 14 *c.* 1930. Pair of polished-steel dress clips, fan-shaped geometric design. 15 *c.* 1938. Silver and rock-crystal brooch, abstract floral design. 16 *c.* 1939. Multicoloured glass stone butterfly brooch. 17 *c.* 1930. Painted-metal novelty brooch, car design set with rhinestones. 18 *c.* 1939. Pair of dress clips, open coffin-shaped plastic body, gold painted clips and trim, shredded bow set with marcasites. 19 *c.* 1935. Pair of metal shoe clips, pierced background set with rhinestones, cabochon fake-emerald terminals.

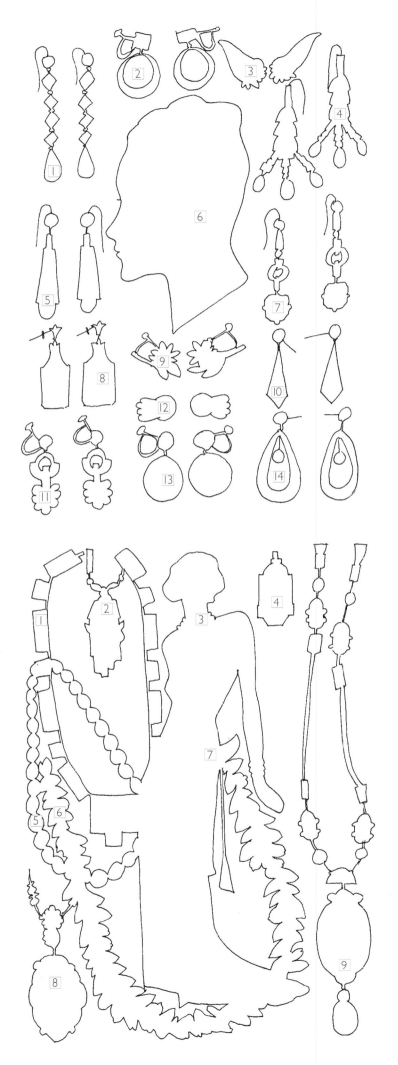

Earrings 1930–1939

1 *c.* 1930. Moulded coloured-glass pendant earrings, small angular beads spaced with tiny gold beads, pear-shaped end drops. 2 *c.* 1930. Silver pendant earrings, hoops set with white paste stones and cushion-shaped fake emeralds, matching studs, screw-type fastenings. 3 *c.* 1930–32. Silver clip-on earrings, shell and flower design set with rhinestones. 4 *c.* 1935. Pendant earrings, graded shaped tears set with diamonds under row of rectangular diamonds, matching pendants supporting engraved teardrop emeralds. In the style of Osterag. 5 *c.* 1930–34. Polished beaten-silver pendant earrings, creased oblong plates supporting oval synthetic sapphires. 6 *c.* 1938. Coloured-plastic clip-on earrings set with white paste stones. 7 *c.* 1930–32. Pendant earrings, rhinestones and synthetic emeralds set in silver. 8 *c.* 1935. Pendant earrings, pierced oblong silver plates set with marcasites, central onyx. 9 *c.* 1930–35. Floral silver-gilt screw-type earrings, set with white paste stones. 10 *c.* 1935. Silver pendant earrings, synthetic ruby and onyx stud above elongated diamond-shaped enamelled pendant. 11 *c.* 1936. Gold pendant earrings, circular and crescent shapes set with brilliant-cut diamonds, matching stud and surround to square diamond pendants. 12 *c.* 1939. Carved-plastic clip-on earrings. 13 *c.* 1939. Plastic earrings, large studs with half-bead spots, matching pendant balls. 14 *c.* 1939. Clear-plastic earrings, bead stud, matching bead drop within open pear-shaped pendant.

Necklaces and Pendants 1930–1939

1 *c.* 1930. Short necklace composed of oblong carved green glass plaques, to imitate jade, spaced by smaller clear amber-coloured glass plaques, silver chain links, settings and fastenings. 2 *c.* 1939. Fine clear-glass necklace, round and oblong beads, supporting a matching asymmetric pendant, with the addition of stylized multicoloured moulded-glass flowers and leaves. 3 *c.* 1938. Short necklace, four rows of graded yellow-gold-coloured glass beads, matching bracelet. 4 *c.* 1934. Oblong oriental-style pendant, polished and engraved-metal border framing carved-jade matrix plaque, floral design. 5 *c.* 1930. Plastic-ivory bead necklace, carved covers in shaded colours over smaller beads, three large central beads, small gold-coloured bead spacers. 6 *c.* 1935. Fine oval glass-bead necklace, threaded with wired transparent glass leaves and textured blown-glass lemons. 7 *c.* 1937. Pendant of asymmetric design, crescent-shaped top, polished and beaten silver, set with plastic half-beads, matching stylized tassels on the ends of two flat chains. 8 *c.* 1935. Silver chain necklace, silver and blue stone bead decoration, floral and foliate support above large pendant, both set with similar stones and matching decoration. 9 *c.* 1935. Long necklace, large oval silver-gilt pendant decorated with fine wire and engraving, clear amber-coloured glass stones mixed with mottled polished stones, matching teardrop to base and links between twisted gold wire necklace.

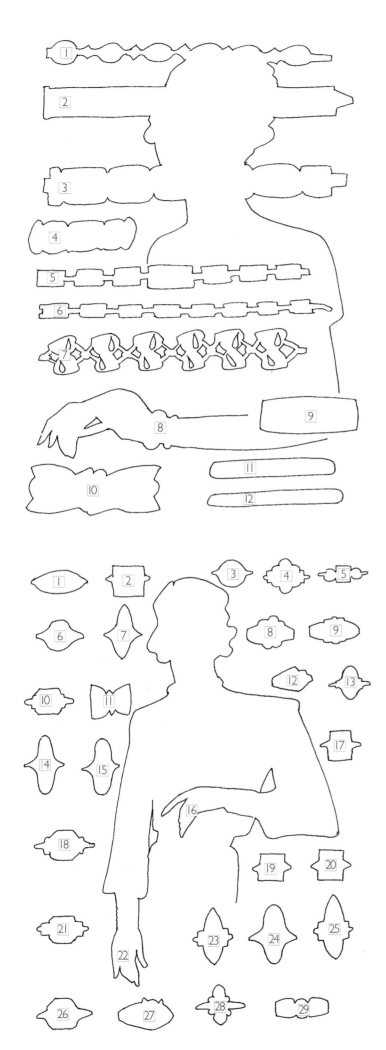

Bracelets and Bangles 1930–1939

1 c. 1930. Bracelet composed of oval plaques, calibré-set with sapphires, diamond-shaped central motif enclosed by diamond-set bands, matching links. 2 c. 1930–35. Bracelet of articulated rectangular panels, set with diamonds and calibré-cut synthetic rubies in geometric formation. 3 c. 1935. Geometric-design bracelet set with baguette- and brilliant-cut diamonds. 4 c. 1935. Carved green plastic bangle, design of tropical leaves and entwined snake, edge-to-edge opening and side-spring hinge. 5 c. 1938. Bracelet composed of a central rectangular plaque decorated with twisted gold wire, large green glass stone, matching smaller stones on each side, small engraved gold-coloured plaques decorated in similar manner, flat links. 6 c. 1939. Eight oblong black onyx plaques edged top and bottom with marcasites, matching articulated double links. 7 c. 1938. Polished-metal bracelet composed of tied ribbon bows, calibré-set with fake sapphires on one side, white paste stones decorate knot and articulated links. 8 c. 1935. Wide green plastic bangle set with tiny white paste stones, edge-to-edge opening, side-spring hinge; narrow polished-copper bangle set with mosaic of coloured stones. 9 c. 1939. Woven gold wire bracelet, width graduated to narrow bow-shaped clasp fastening on centre-front. 10 c. 1935. Moulded ivory-coloured plastic bangle, draped and twisted design, opening under central knot, back-spring hinge. 11 c. 1935. Silver-coloured metal bangle set with coloured and white paste stones, side-clip opening. 12 c. 1938. Narrow flexible plastic bangle set with multicoloured glass stones.

Rings 1930–1939

1 c. 1930. Cabochon opals, diamond surround. 2 c. 1933. Checkerboard design, composed of sapphires and diamonds. 3 c. 1935. Large diamond set within diamond border. 4 c. 1935. Rectangular emerald set within diamond border, matching shoulders. 5 c. 1930. Rectangular sapphire, diamond-set shoulders. 6 c. 1935. Cabochon stone set in silver, engraved shoulders. 7 c. 1937. Marquise diamond, diamond-set shoulders. 8 c. 1935. Scroll design set with diamonds, outer border of cabochon rubies and small diamonds. 9 c. 1936. Rectangular emerald, deep diamond-set shoulders. 10 c. 1934. Rectangular sapphire, diamond shoulders. 11 c. 1938. Marquise-shaped diamond set in gold bow-shaped mount. 12 c. 1939. Deep gold-coloured metal band, architectural detail set with fake rubies. 13 c. 1935. Coloured stone set within pierced oval silver mount. 14 c. 1935. Rectangular stone set within marquise-shaped metal mount. 15 c. 1930. Pierced marquise-shaped ring set with marcasites. 16 c. 1937. Oval cabochon emerald. 17 c. 1935. Rectangular plaque set with paste sapphires and emeralds against a white paste background. 18 c. 1935. Diamond cluster ring, radiating rows of calibré-cut emeralds. 19 c. 1938. Rectangular ruby, diamond surround. 20 c. 1938. Pierced plaque, central sapphire, diamond surround. 21 c. 1939. Rectangular diamond, matching step shoulders. 22 c. 1937. Marquise-shaped stone, paste shoulders. 23 c. 1935–39. Marquise-shaped glass stone, step shoulders. 24 c. 1935–39. Pierced marquise-shaped set with coloured stones. 25 c. 1935–39. Marquise-shaped rock crystal, central diamond, diamond surround and shoulders. 26 c. 1935. Octagonal ring set with cabochon stone. 27 c. 1939. Panther ring set with diamonds, onyx and emeralds. In the style of Cartier. 28 c. 1930. Cabochon stones set in gold wire frame. 29 c. 1939. Split two-colour gold band, set with synthetic cabochon ruby bead.

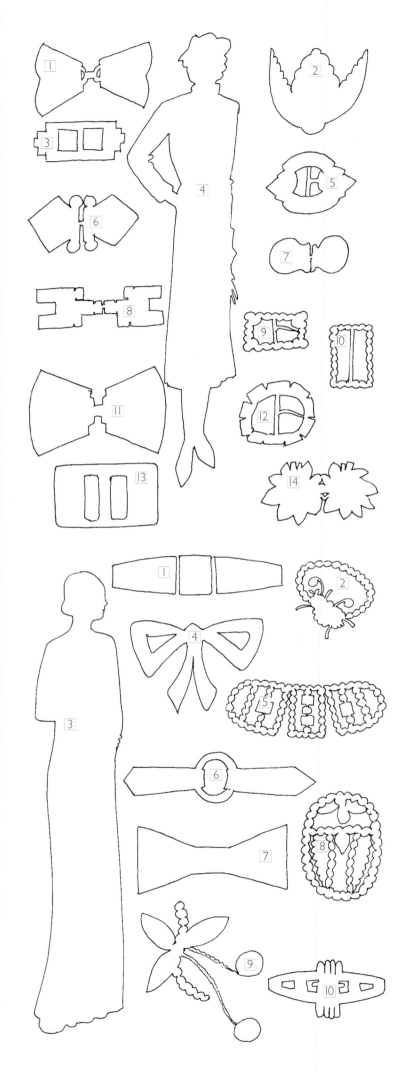

Buckles and Clasps 1930–1939

1 c. 1935. Fan-shaped gold-washed-brass cape clasp, stamped design of birds, flowers and leaves. 2 c. 1930–34. Gold-painted brass-filigree belt clasp, bird design, set with cabochon turquoise stones. 3 c. 1930. Narrow gold-washed-brass dress buckle, plastic side panels, matching pattern of top and bottom bars, gold painted highlights. 4 c. 1937. Half-moon-shaped polished-brass clasp, leather-covered connector, leather belt, matching set of buttons. 5 c. 1935. Oval dress buckle, patterned silk panels under clear plastic, contrast-colour trim, single-prong fastener. 6 c. 1930. Moulded coloured-glass dress clasp prong-mounted in silver, two moulded clear-glass spacers. 7 c. 1939. Chromium-plated metal belt clasp, flat circular design decorated with triangular plastic stones facing away from folded edges of centre. 8 c. 1930. Clear moulded-glass dress clasp, rectangular brick design with small square spacers, fine paste-set end bars. 9 c. 1930. Rectangular brass dress buckle with prong-set rhinestones. 10 c. 1935. Oblong brass dress buckle with prong-set rhinestones and fake cabochon emeralds. 11 c. 1935–39. Fan-shaped plastic belt clasp, gold-coloured metal trim set with plastic half-beads in matching colour. 12 c. 1935. Brass belt-buckle, prong-set clear and coloured moulded-glass stones. 13 c. 1935–39. Rectangular plastic coat buckle, carved stripes highlighted with gold paint. 14 c. 1930. Gold-washed-brass dress clasp, design of pierced leaves and bezel-set moulded coloured-glass stones.

Dress Ornaments 1930–1939

1 c. 1930. Three-piece belt ornament, rectangular central panel set with large central white paste stone and twisted gold-coloured wire decoration, prong-set white paste stone surround, matching graduated side panels. 2 c. 1935–39. Lapel ornament, coloured and clear paste stone fly-mounted on semicircular wreath of prong-set paste stones, gold-coloured bead spacers. 3 c. 1934. Bias-cut satin evening dress with large paste butterfly set on base of low back neckline. 4 c. 1935–39. Articulated bow-knot dress ornament, prong-set white paste stones within gold-coloured metal frame. 5 c. 1930. Three-piece belt ornament, rectangular central panel, two large paste stones set within rectangular gold-coloured wire frames, paste stone surround, matching semicircular side panels, hinges between panels on upper rod. 6 c. 1935. Mock belt and oval buckle beaded in black and white. 7 c. 1937–39. Rigid gold wire bow-shaped dress ornament, decorated with lines of prong-set white paste stones and gold bead spacers. 8 c. 1930. Gold-coloured metal open dress ornament, twisted wire and bead decoration, prong-set pale-coloured paste stones, matching oval surround. 9 c. 1939. Evening dress ornament of gold-coloured wire construction, leaf spray and berry design, prong-set with white paste stones. 10 c. 1930–35. Articulated dress or belt ornament, two matching open side panels set with marcasites and fake cushion-shaped emeralds, hinges each side of vertical central bars.

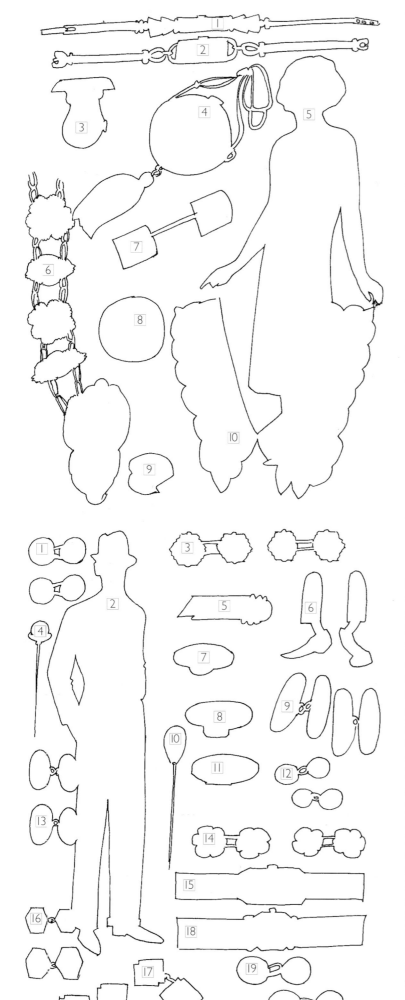

Miscellaneous Jewelry and Jewelled Pieces 1920–1939

1 *c.* 1935–39. Platinum bracelet watch, oblong case set with baguette-cut diamonds, fan-shaped shoulders set with brilliant- and baguette-cut diamonds, fine mesh strap with adjustable fastening. 2 *c.* 1920–25. Platinum bracelet watch, oblong case and hinged cover set with diamonds, matching hemispherical shoulders and rope-pattern bracelet, adjustable fastening. 3 *c.* 1939. Circular platinum lapel watch, case set with brilliant-cut diamonds, row of graded baguette diamonds from pin to top of watch face. 4 *c.* 1930–36. Jade-look plastic powder compact set with circular panel of rhinestones, matching clasp fastening and beads threaded onto silk card handle, silk tassel on base. 5 *c.* 1923. Fine silk-georgette evening dress with embroidered panels of glass beads and sequins. 6 *c.* 1925. Silver belt composed of fine openwork plaques, linked together with chain, each plaque set with multicoloured cabochon stones and hand-painted with coloured enamels. 7 *c.* 1935. Plastic hat ornament set with clear glass stones, metal linking pin. 8 *c.* 1929. Silver-coloured metal powder compact, design of dragonflies enamelled onto lid. 9 *c.* 1929. Multicoloured plastic scarf-ring set with tiny clear glass stones. 10 *c.* 1930. Silk collar covered with pattern of coloured-glass bugle beads.

Men's Jewelry 1920–1939

1 *c.* 1920–25. Dark-grey mother-of-pearl cufflinks, centre of each circular plaque decorated with crossed bars set with diamonds, enamelled outer border with diamond detail. 2 *c.* 1935–39. Gold bar tie pin, square gold cufflinks set in centre with synthetic ruby. 3 *c.* 1930. Carved frosted-rock-crystal cufflinks, stepped design overlaid with diamond-set band. 4 *c.* 1920–25. Gold stickpin, cabochon sapphire set inside engraved collar of leaves. 5 *c.* 1934. Silver tie clip. In the style of Theodor Fahrner. 6 *c.* 1930. Silver cufflinks with enamelled abstract design, solid bar connections. In the style of Theodor Fahrner. 7 *c.* 1936. Silver ring, large cabochon stone, carved shoulders. In the style of Theodor Fahrner. 8 *c.* 1936. Silver ring, cushion-shaped onyx, raised and carved shoulders. In the style of Theodor Fahrner. 9 *c.* 1930–39. Oval lapis lazuli cabochon stones set in gold, matching chain links. 10 *c.* 1920. Marbled-glass top to gold stickpin. 11 *c.* 1935–39. Gold ring, flat square mottled stone, pierced shoulder. 12 *c.* 1920–29. Gold cufflinks composed of matching cabochon-cut rubies, oval link connections. 13 *c.* 1920–29. Gold-coloured metal cufflinks, enamelled oval plaques, sailing-ship design. 14 *c.* 1920–25. Gold floral cufflinks, centrally set ruby. 15 *c.* 1935. Chrome wristwatch, luminous numerals and hands, stitched leather strap. 16 *c.* 1925–30. Gold octagonal cufflinks, onyx plaques with centrally set diamond. 17 *c.* 1925–30. Square gold cufflinks, raised central diamonds, stepped border. 18 *c.* 1935. Gold wristwatch, octagonal shape, textured leather strap. 19 *c.* 1930–35. Gold cufflinks, one plaque set with large mother-of-pearl centre, surround of sapphires, the other of mother-of-pearl with small inner circle of sapphires.

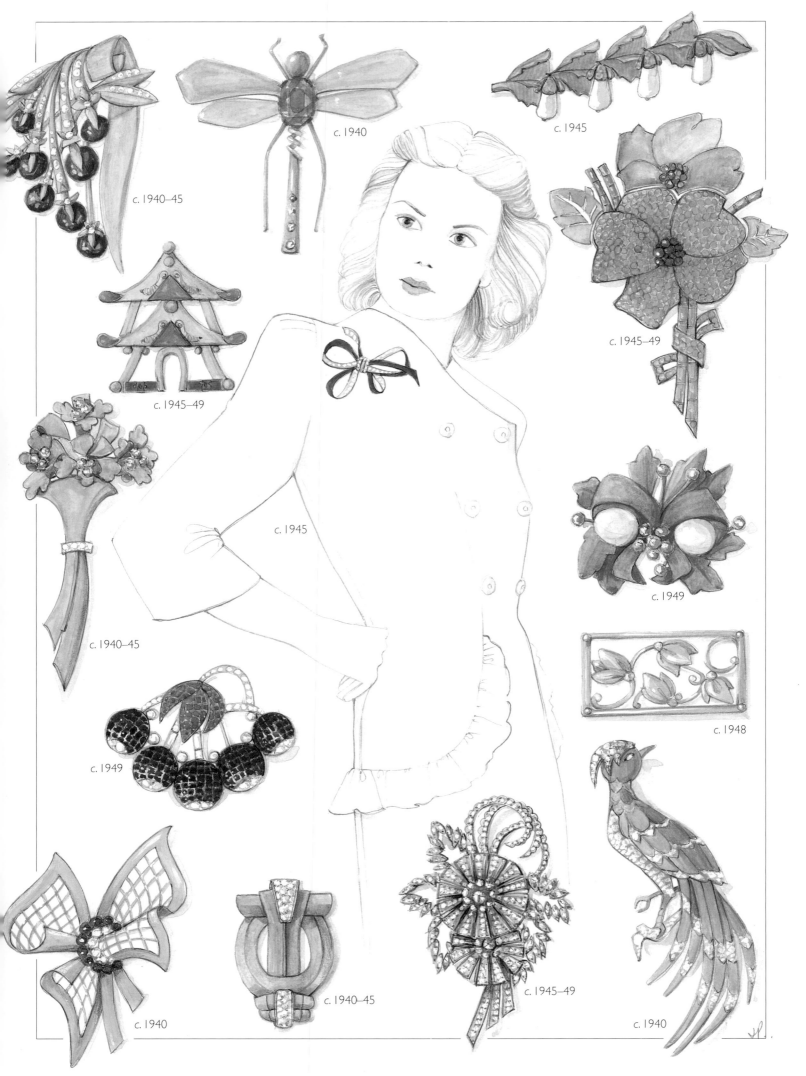

c. 1940–45

c. 1940

c. 1945

c. 1945–49

c. 1945–49

c. 1940–45

c. 1945

c. 1949

c. 1948

c. 1949

c. 1940

c. 1940–45

c. 1945–49

c. 1940

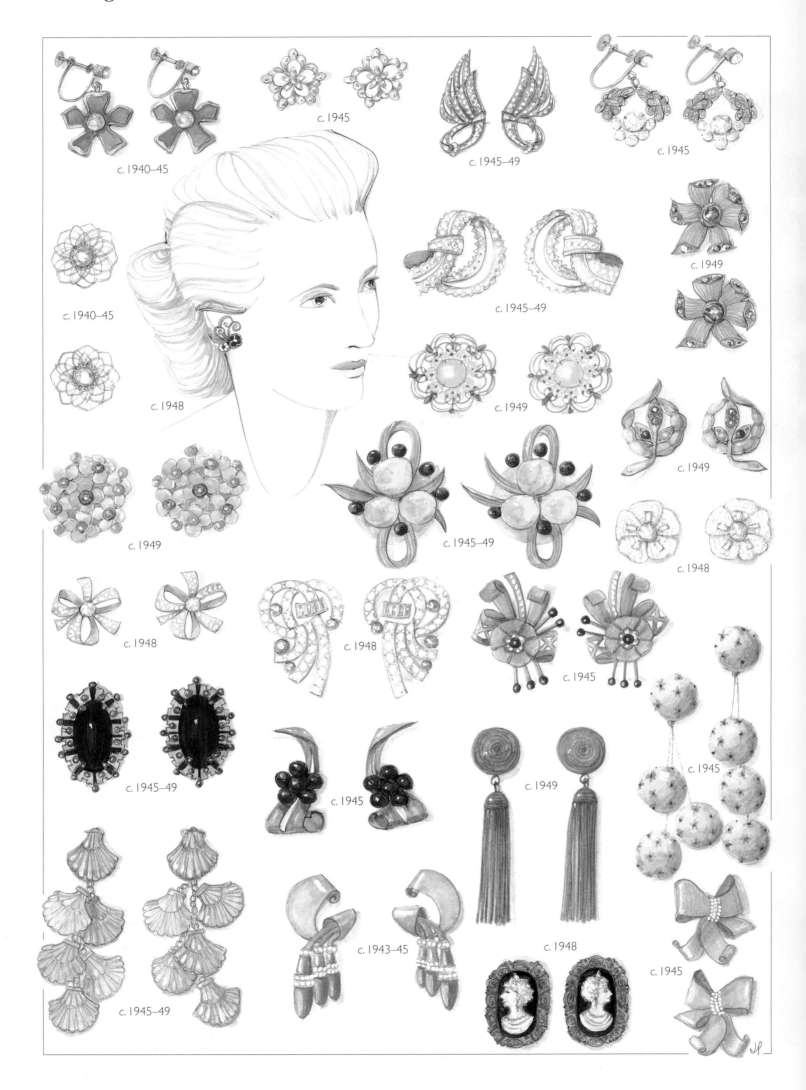

c. 1940–45

c. 1945

c. 1945–49

c. 1945

c. 1940–45

c. 1945–49

c. 1949

c. 1948

c. 1949

c. 1949

c. 1945–49

c. 1949

c. 1948

c. 1949

c. 1948

c. 1948

c. 1945

c. 1948

c. 1945

c. 1945–49

c. 1945

c. 1949

c. 1945

c. 1945–49

c. 1943–45

c. 1948

c. 1945

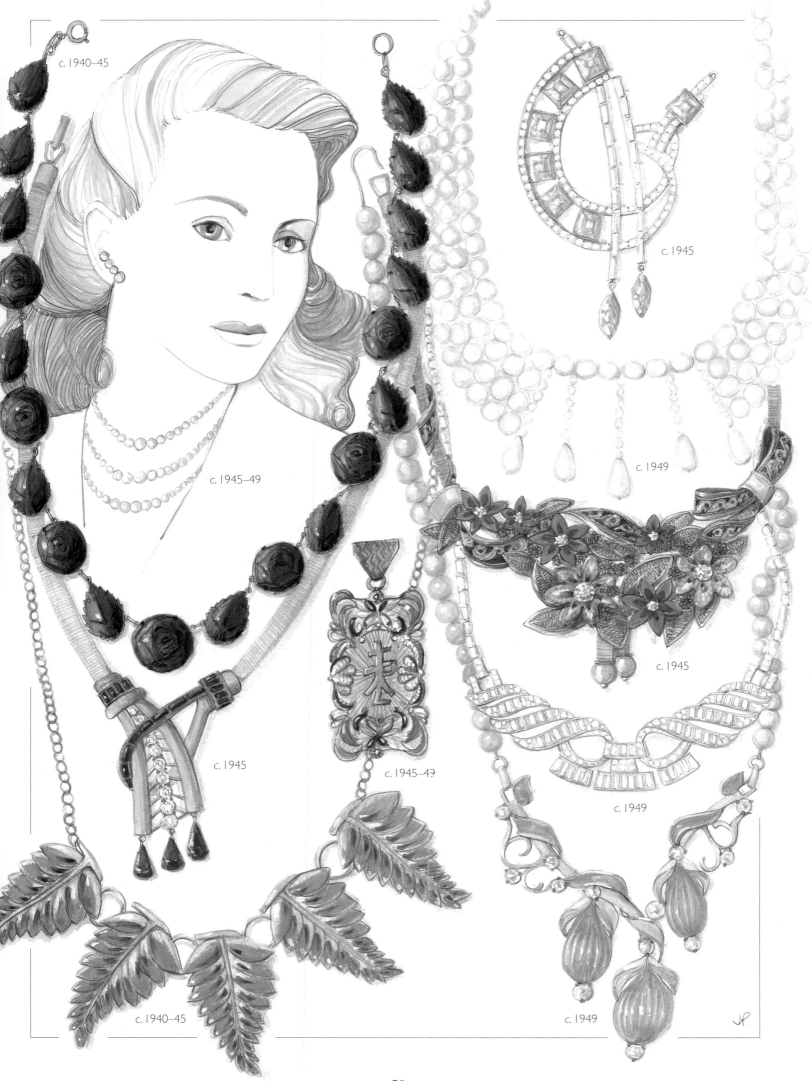

c. 1940–45

c. 1945

c. 1945–49

c. 1949

c. 1945

c. 1945–49

c. 1945

c. 1949

c. 1940–45

c. 1949

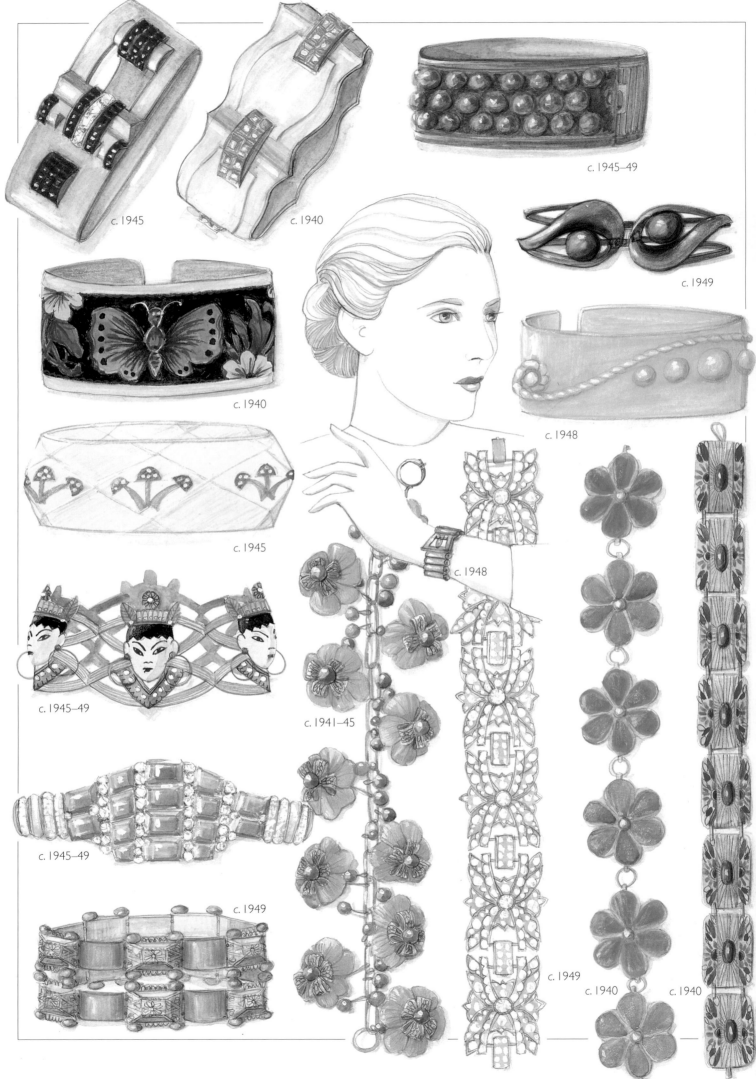

c. 1945

c. 1940

c. 1945–49

c. 1949

c. 1940

c. 1948

c. 1945

c. 1948

c. 1945–49

c. 1941–45

c. 1949

c. 1945–49

c. 1949

c. 1940

c. 1940

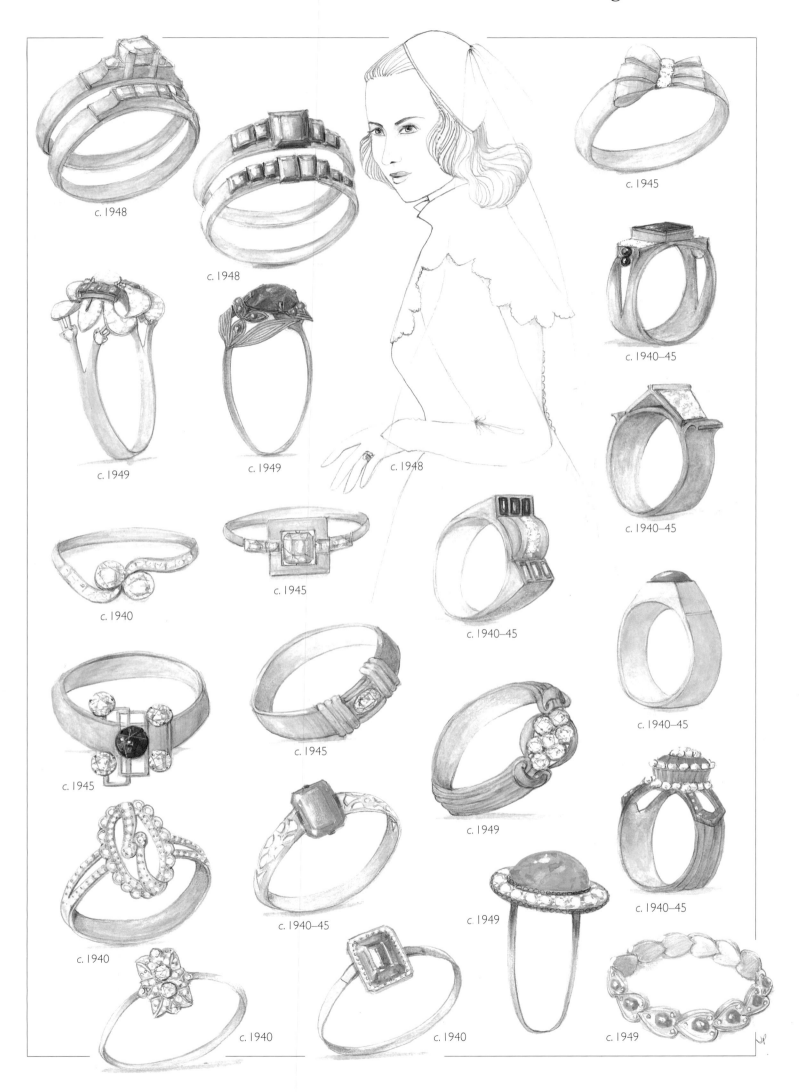

c. 1948

c. 1948

c. 1945

c. 1940–45

c. 1949

c. 1949

c. 1948

c. 1940–45

c. 1940

c. 1945

c. 1940–45

c. 1940–45

c. 1945

c. 1945

c. 1949

c. 1940–45

c. 1940

c. 1940–45

c. 1949

c. 1940

c. 1940

c. 1949

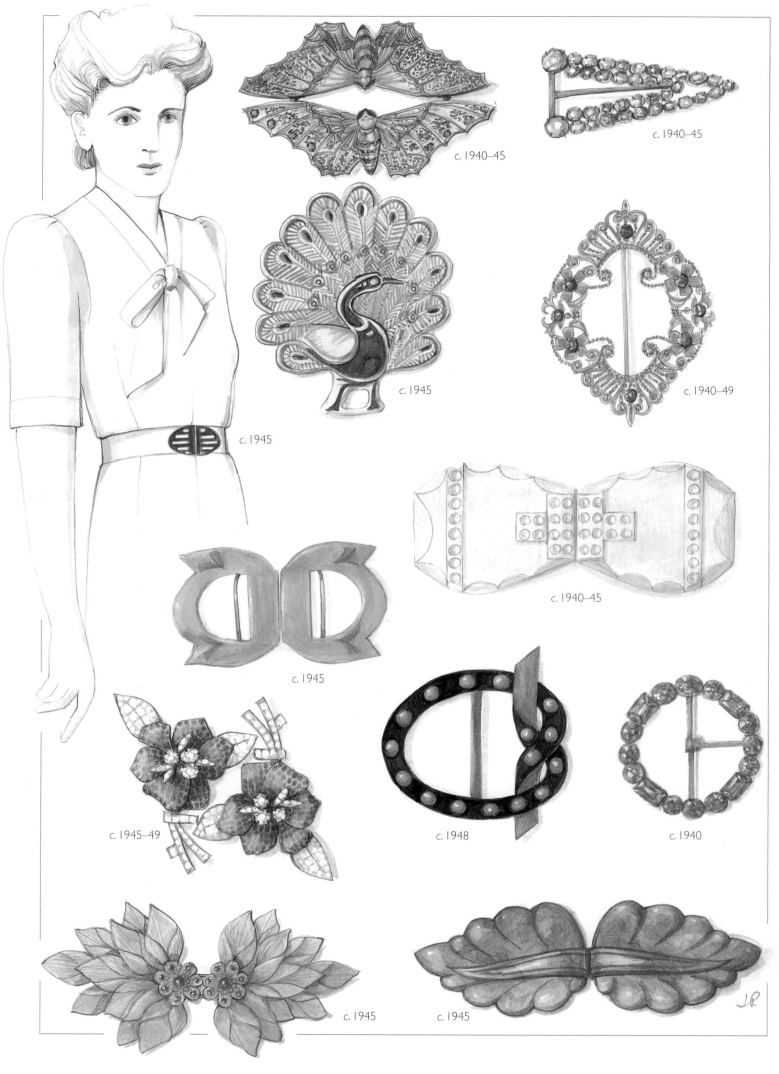

c. 1940–45

c. 1940–45

c. 1945

c. 1940–49

c. 1945

c. 1940–45

c. 1945

c. 1945–49

c. 1948

c. 1940

c. 1945

c. 1945

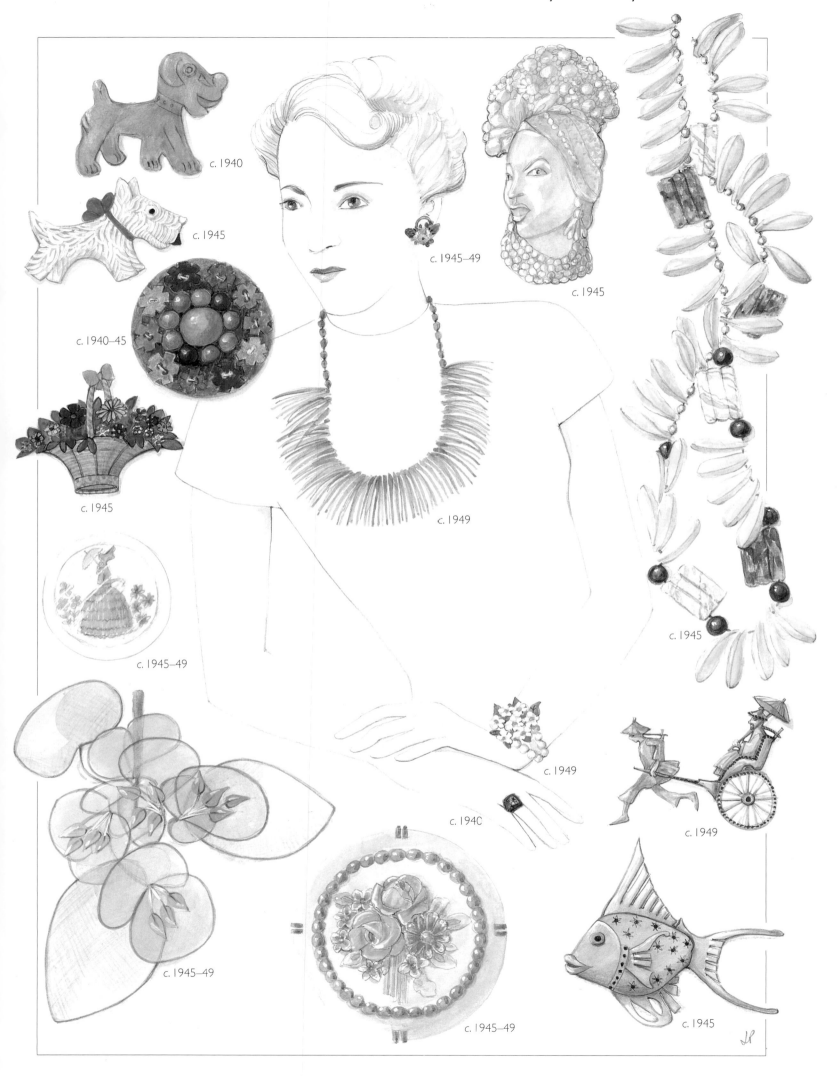

c. 1940

c. 1945

c. 1940–45

c. 1945

c. 1945–49

c. 1945–49

c. 1945–49

c. 1945–49

c. 1945–49

c. 1940

c. 1945

c. 1945

c. 1949

c. 1949

c. 1949

c. 1945

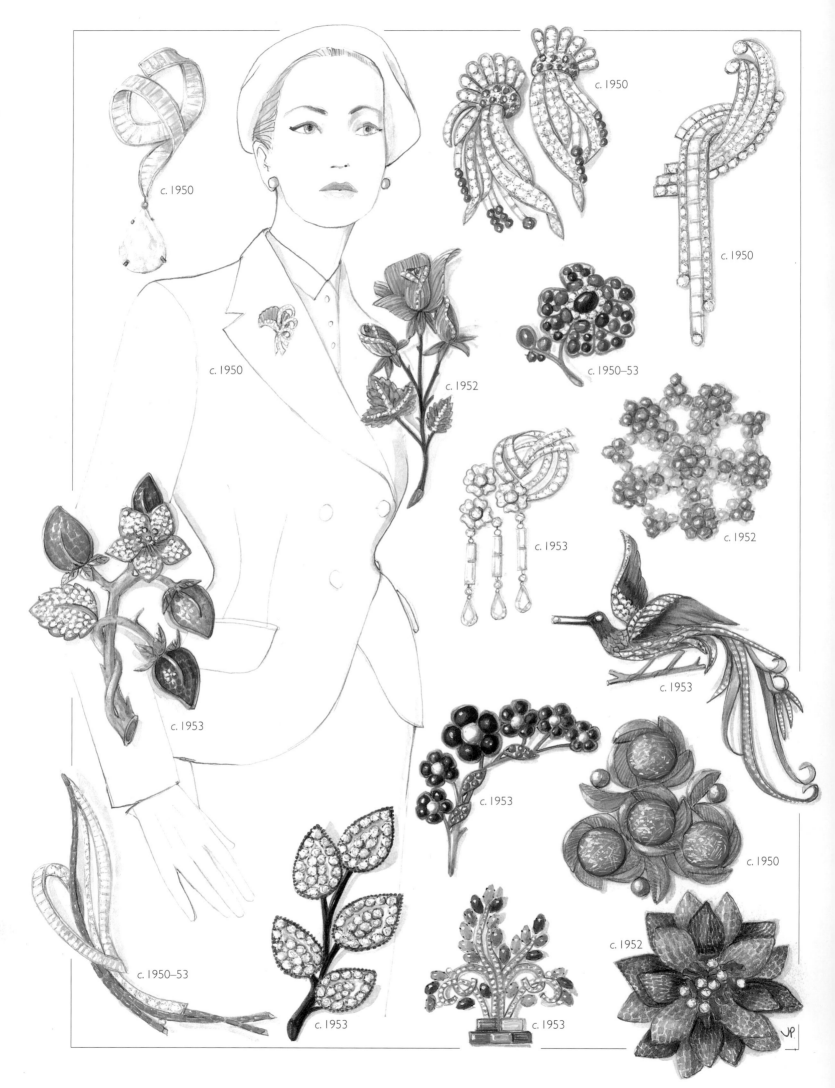

c. 1950

c. 1950

c. 1950

c. 1950

c. 1952

c. 1950–53

c. 1952

c. 1953

c. 1953

c. 1953

c. 1953

c. 1953

c. 1950

c. 1950–53

c. 1953

c. 1953

c. 1952

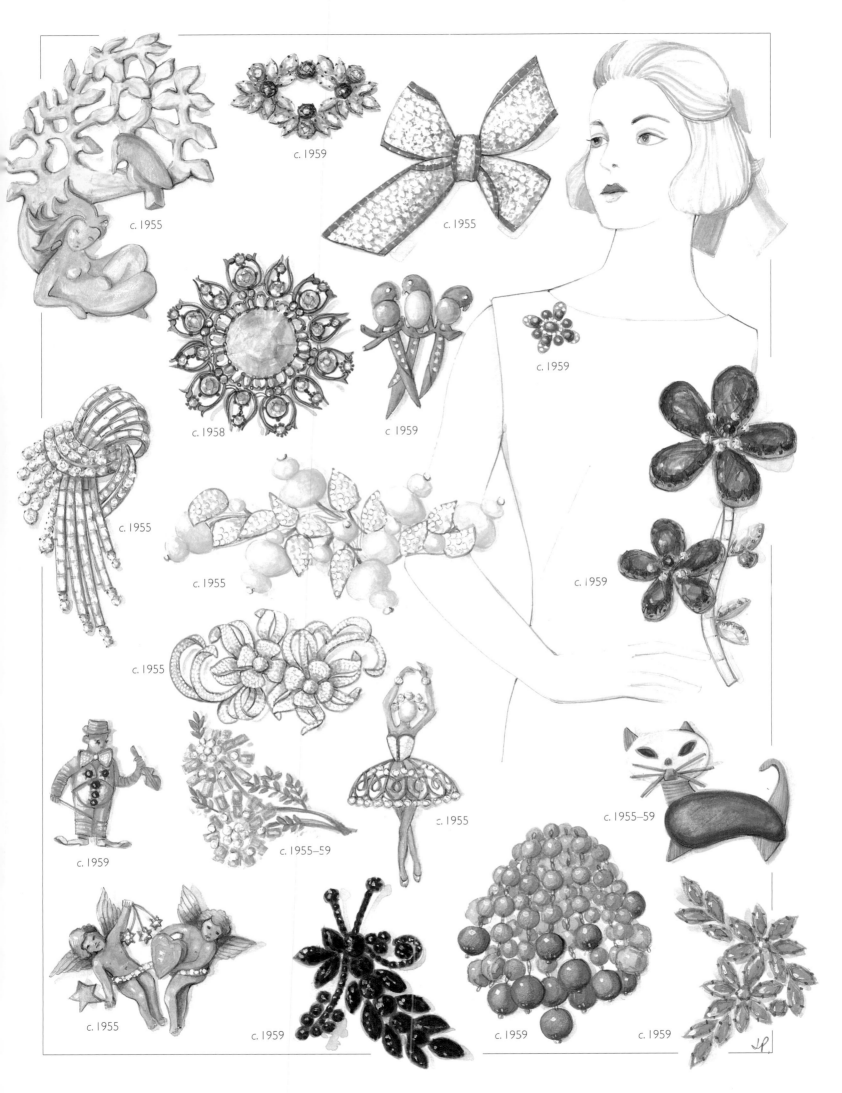

c. 1959

c. 1955

c. 1955

c. 1958

c 1959

c. 1959

c. 1955

c. 1955

c. 1959

c. 1955

c. 1959

c. 1955

c. 1955–59

c. 1955

c. 1955–59

c. 1955

c. 1959

c. 1959

c. 1959

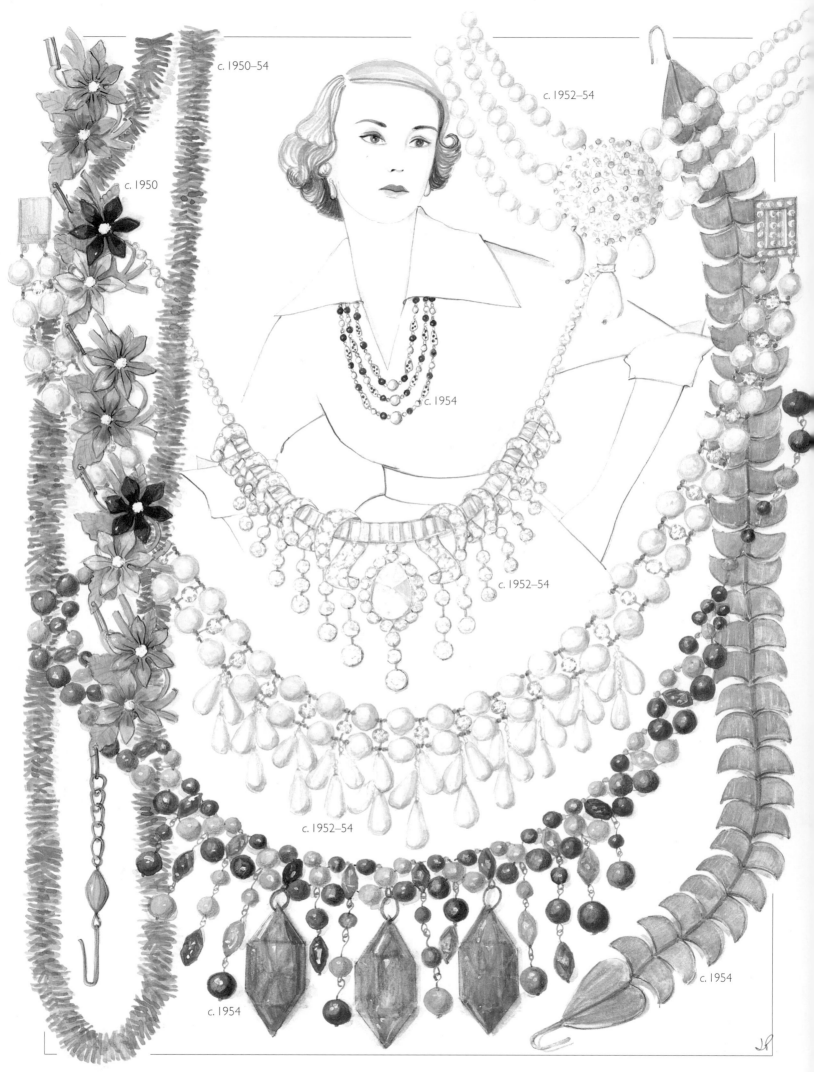

c. 1950–54

c. 1950

c. 1952–54

c. 1954

c. 1952–54

c. 1952–54

c. 1954

c. 1954

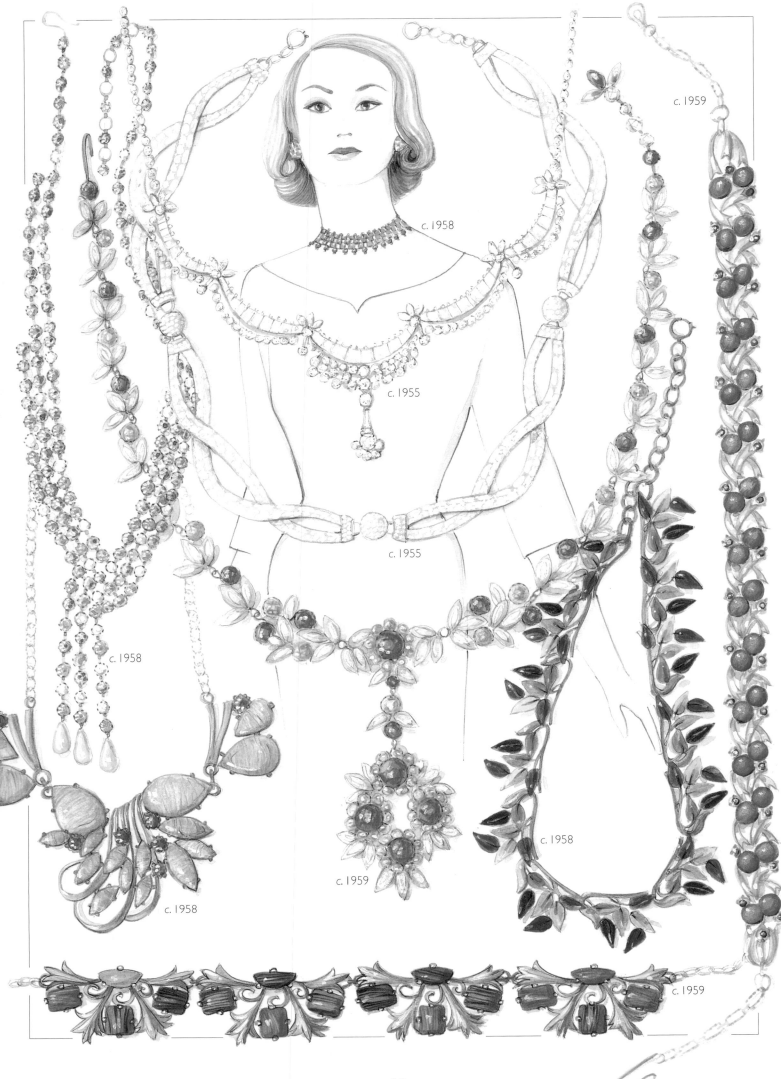

c. 1959

c. 1958

c. 1955

c. 1955

c. 1958

c. 1958

c. 1958

c. 1959

c. 1958

c. 1959

Bracelets and Bangles 1950–1959

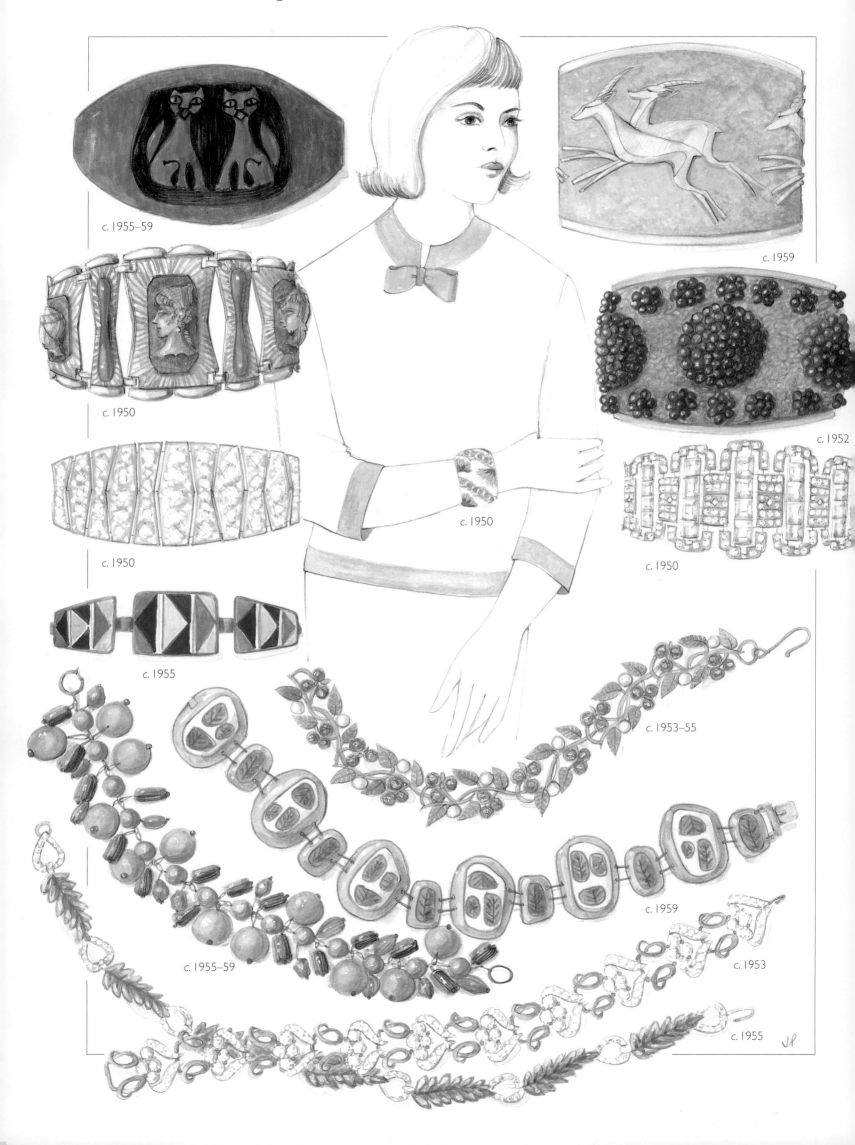

c. 1955–59

c. 1959

c. 1950

c. 1950

c. 1950

c. 1952

c. 1950

c. 1955

c. 1953–55

c. 1959

c. 1955–59

c. 1953

c. 1955

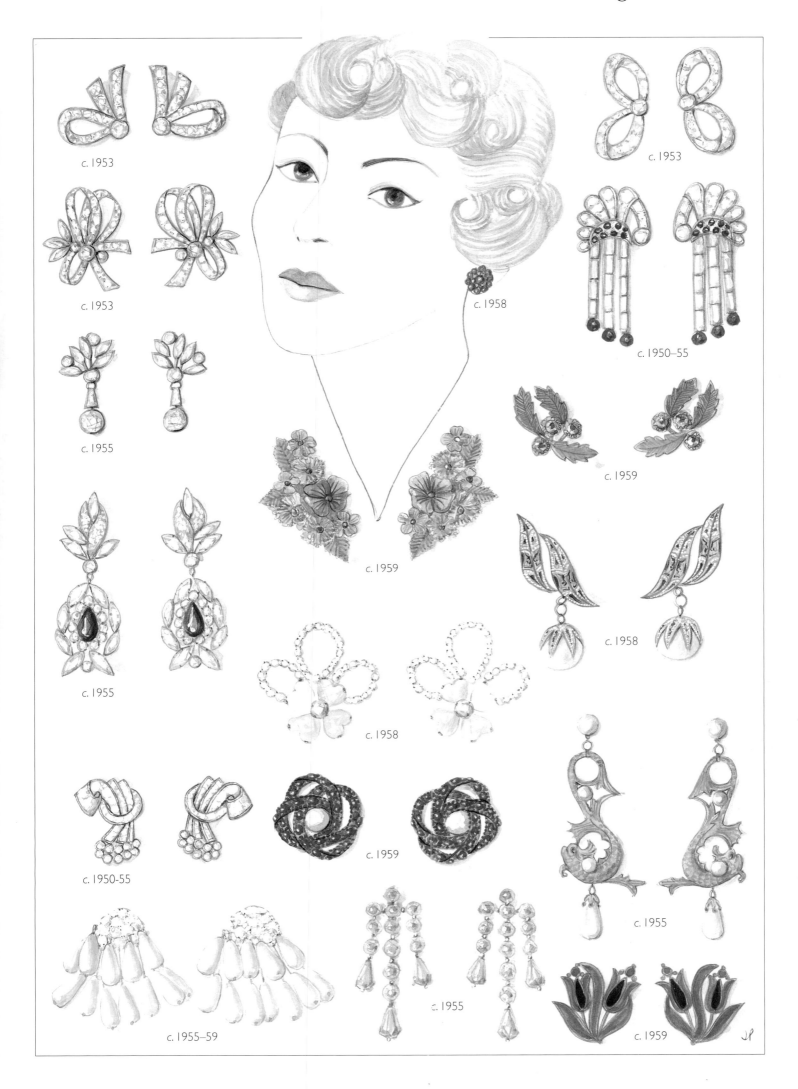

c. 1953

c. 1953

c. 1953

c. 1958

c. 1950–55

c. 1955

c. 1959

c. 1959

c. 1955

c. 1958

c. 1958

c. 1950-55

c. 1959

c. 1955

c. 1955–59

c. 1955

c. 1959

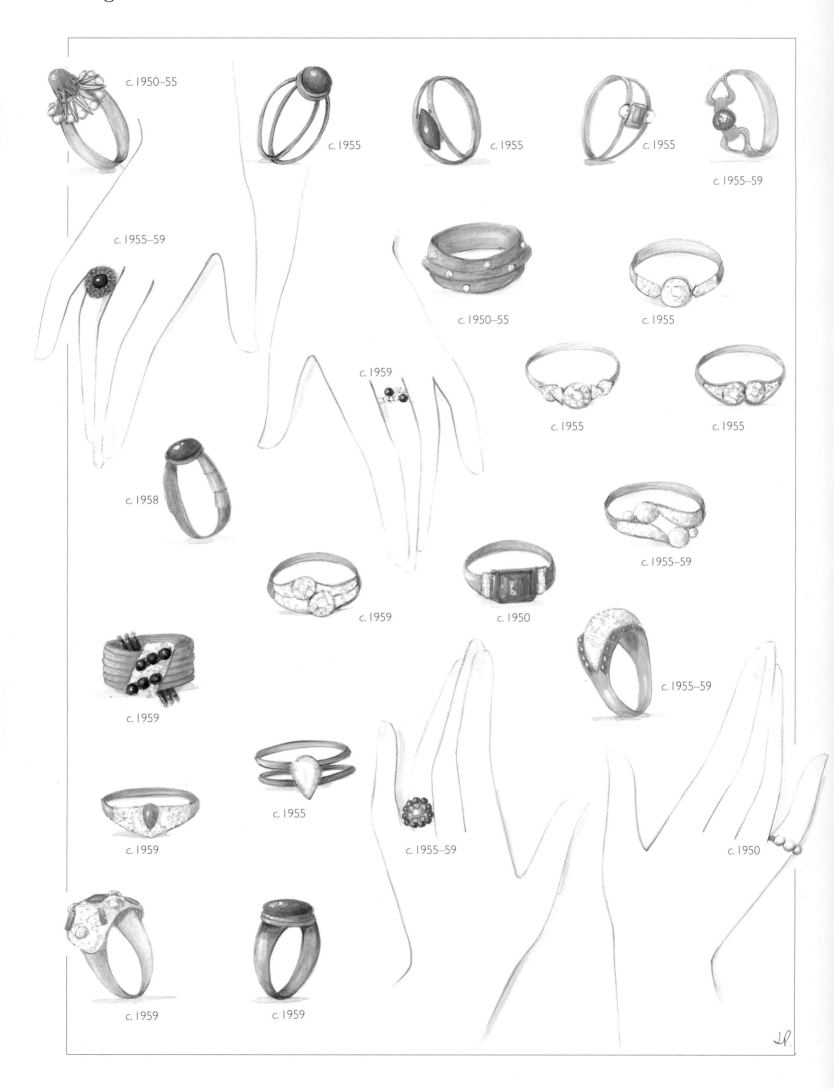

c. 1950–55

c. 1955

c. 1955

c. 1955

c. 1955–59

c. 1955–59

c. 1950–55

c. 1955

c. 1959

c. 1955

c. 1955

c. 1958

c. 1955–59

c. 1959

c. 1950

c. 1959

c. 1955–59

c. 1959

c. 1955

c. 1955–59

c. 1950

c. 1959

c. 1959

Miscellaneous Jewelry and Jewelled Pieces 1940–1959

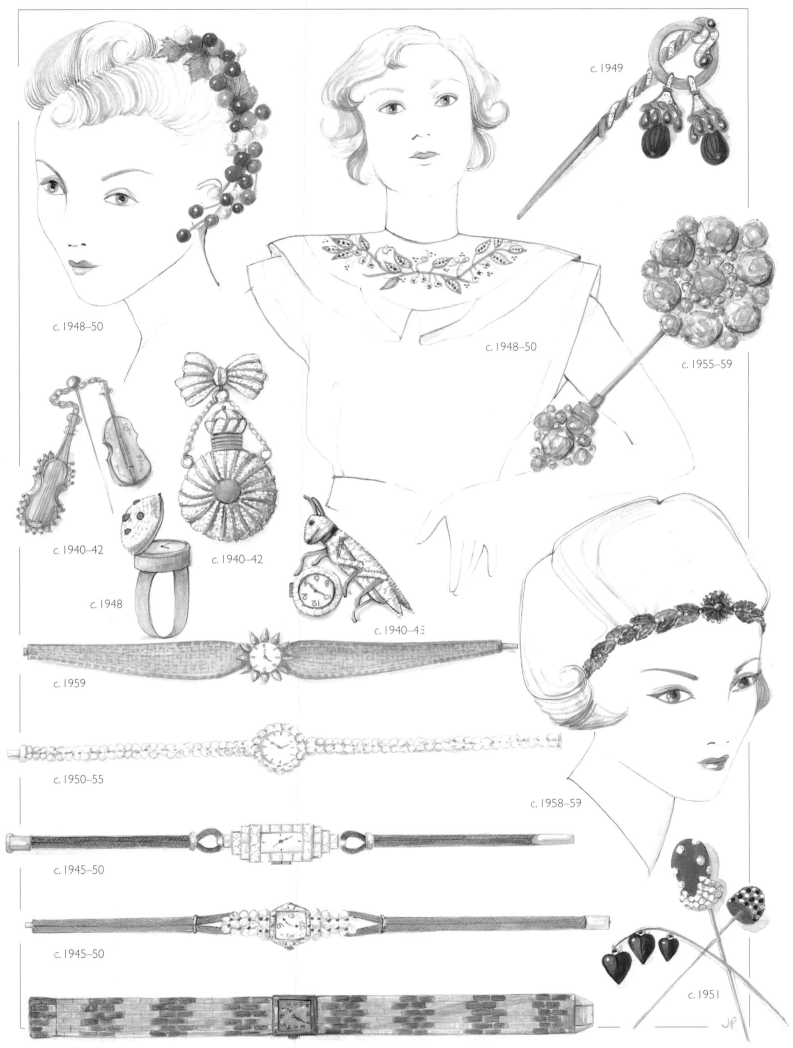

c. 1949

c. 1948–50

c. 1948–50

c. 1955–59

c. 1940–42

c. 1940–42

c. 1948

c. 1940–43

c. 1959

c. 1958–59

c. 1950–55

c. 1945–50

c. 1945–50

c. 1951

c. 1940–45

Men's Jewelry 1940–1959

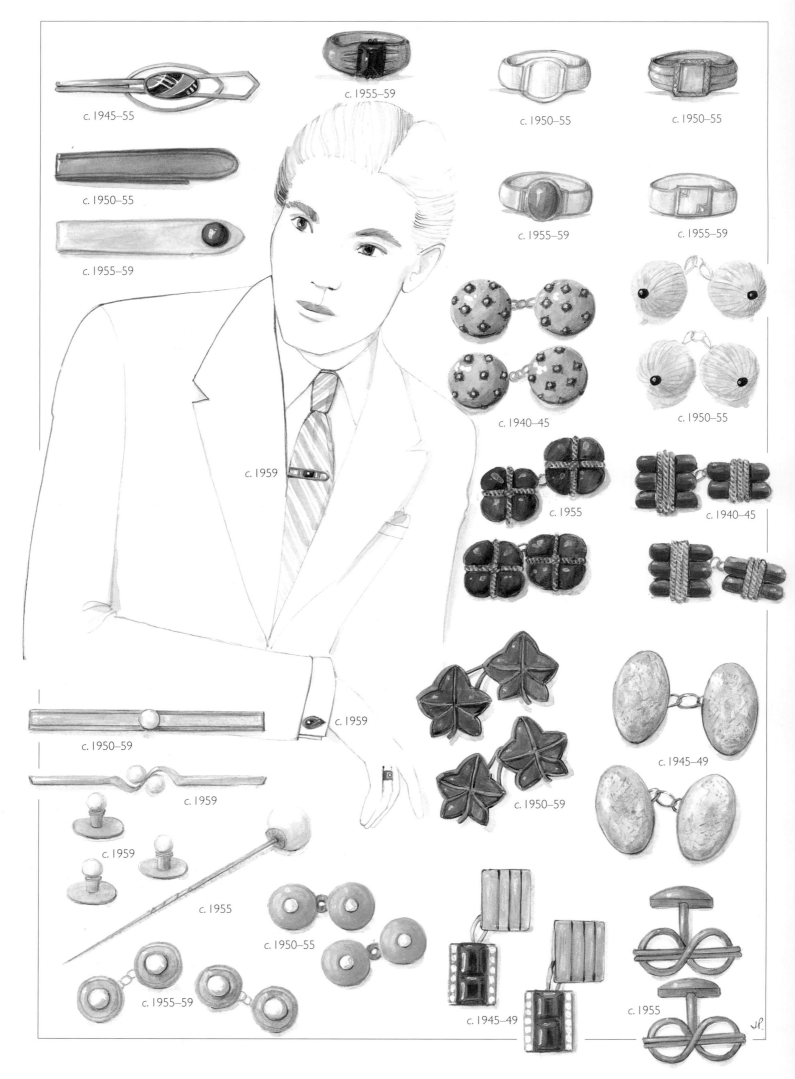

c. 1945–55

c. 1955–59

c. 1950–55

c. 1950–55

c. 1950–55

c. 1955–59

c. 1955–59

c. 1959

c. 1940–45

c. 1950–55

c. 1955

c. 1940–45

c. 1950–59

c. 1959

c. 1945–49

c. 1959

c. 1959

c. 1950–59

c. 1955

c. 1950–55

c. 1955–59

c. 1945–49

c. 1955

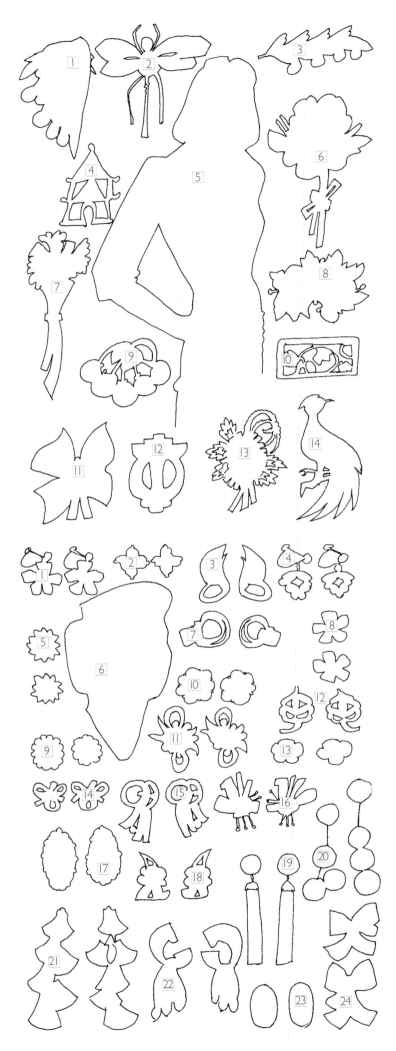

Brooches and Clips 1940–1949

1 c. 1940–45. Polished-brass dress clip, flat moulded-glass beads representing stylized fruit, stems and leaves set with clear stones. 2 c. 1940. Polished-brass dragonfly brooch, large coloured cut-glass stone body, matching stones at base of tail. 3 c. 1945. Gilded-metal bar brooch, design of leaves, touched with enamel, long fake pearl drop flowers. 4 c. 1945–49. Gold painted metal pagoda brooch, set with triangular fake-jade stones, matching stones at the end of gable roofs, red stones each side arched doorway. 5 c. 1945. Knotted and looped bow brooch, enamelled in deep pink on underside, and set with clear paste stones on top. 6 c. 1945–49. Floral brooch, polished-brass flower and leaves set behind similar flower set with small turquoise stones and a centre of coral stones. 7 c. 1940–45. Polished-brass flower spray brooch, coloured paste stones and scalloped leaves, the tie set with white paste stones. 8 c. 1949. Polished-copper brooch, bow and leaf design, white blown-glass beads set inside bow loops. 9 c. 1949. Silver brooch, berries and leaves set with flat synthetic diamonds, rubies and emeralds. 10 c. 1948. Rectangular polished-silver brooch, openwork design of flowers and stems. In the style of Georg Jensen. 11 c. 1940. Silver bow brooch, openwork mesh design, knot of rubies and diamonds. 12 c. 1940–45. Two-colour gold scroll-design dress clip, pavé-set diamond detail to intersecting tapered band. 13 c. 1945–49. Floral spray marcasite brooch. 14 c. 1940. Jay brooch gilded in two colours, details set with white paste stones. In the style of Marcel Boucher Ltd.

Earrings 1940–1949

1 c. 1940–45. Floral pendant earrings, coloured-glass stones set in centre of plastic petals, screw fasteners. 2 c. 1945. Floral marcasite clip-on earrings. 3 c. 1945–49. Feather-design marcasite clip-on earrings. 4 c. 1945. Silver pendant earrings, wreath design set with white paste stones, screw fasteners. 5 c. 1940–45. Gold wire clip-on earrings, floral design, coloured paste stone set in centre. 6 c. 1948. Gold-plated clip-on earrings, flower spray design, set with coloured stones. 7 c. 1945–49. Silver and marcasite clip-on earrings, pierced loop design. 8 c. 1949. Gold-plated clip-on earrings, central coloured stone, matching stones on outer edges. 9 c. 1949. Clip-on earrings, plastic flowers with coloured-glass centres, flat circular base. 10 c. 1949. Gold wire clip-on earrings, central cabochon stone, similar surround. 11 c. 1945–49. Clip-on earrings, still life of plastic berries and gilt leaves, flat circular base. 12 c. 1949. Wreath-design clip-on earrings, central leaves set with coloured stones. 13 c. 1948. Floral clip-on platinum earrings set with diamonds. 14 c. 1948. Ribbon-bow clip-on platinum earrings set with diamonds. 15 c. 1948. Clip-on platinum earrings, interlocked open circles and ribbon ends set with diamonds and sapphires. 16 c. 1945. Gold earrings, floral design against pierced ribbons, set with cabochon rubies and diamonds. In the style of Cartier. 17 c. 1945–49. Polished-wood earrings, gold painted mount. 18 c. 1945. Gold leaf-shaped earrings set with a cluster of garnets. 19 c. 1949. Polished-copper earrings, engraved studs, matching caps to pendant tassels. 20 c. 1945. Pendant earrings, gold balls set with tiny rubies. In the style of Van Cleef & Arpels. 21 c. 1945–49. Two-colour gold-shell-design pendant earrings. 22 c. 1943–45. Gold earrings, diamond and cabochon sapphire pendants. In the style of Boucheron. 23 c. 1948. Plastic cameo earrings, gold painted surround. 24 c. 1945. Gold ribbon-bow earrings, knot set with diamonds. In the style of Mauboussin.

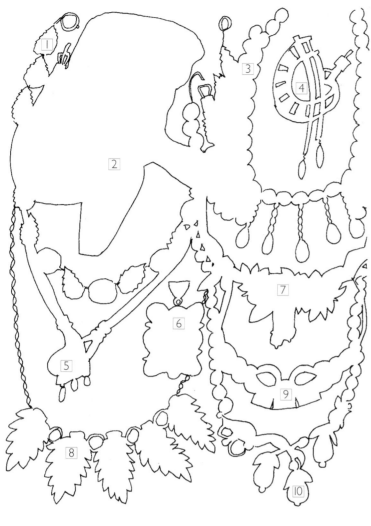

Necklaces and Pendants 1940–1949

1 *c.* 1940–45. Short carved red plastic necklace, floral and foliate design, silver links and fastenings. 2 *c.* 1945–49. Three rows of graded fake pearls, matching clip earrings. 3 *c.* 1949. Short four-strand fake-pearl collar, linked at front by single row of pearls, pear-shaped droplets suspended from tiny fake-pearl strands. 4 *c.* 1945. Asymmetric pendant, cushion-shaped synthetic sapphires set within diamond borders, two matching pendants suspended under bars of pavé-set diamonds. 5 *c.* 1945. Short gold necklace, flexible chain, linked front detail set with rubies and diamonds, matching ruby pendants. 6 *c.* 1945–49. Gold-coloured metal pendant, oriental design highlighted with multicoloured enamels. 7 *c.* 1945. Gold necklace, flexible chain, asymmetric half-wreath of enamelled flowers set with brilliant-cut diamonds, engraved leaves, matching loops of ribbon. 8 *c.* 1940–45. Large gold-coloured metal leaves touched with brightly coloured enamel, linked by large rings, fine chain back. 9 *c.* 1949. Short platinum necklace balanced architectural design set with brilliant- and baguette-cut diamonds, matching back chain. 10 *c.* 1949. Shiny gold-plated beads supporting asymmetric foliate-design pendant, branches swathed in enamelled ribbon and set with pale coloured-glass stones, matching pear-shaped carved-plastic berries.

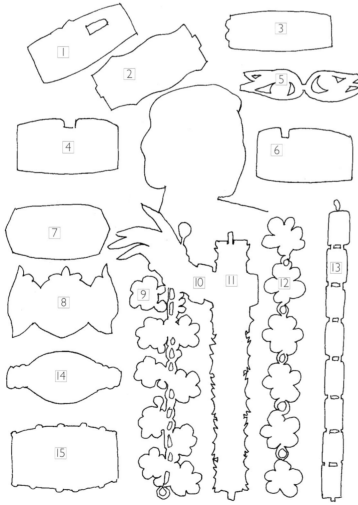

Bracelets and Bangles 1940–1949

1 *c.* 1945. Asymmetric-design gold bangle, front-hinged fastening, set with line of brilliant-cut diamonds bordered by channel-set rubies, matching decoration to shoulders. 2 *c.* 1940. Gold bangle, designed as a hinged cuff with a scalloped edge, set with bands of channel-set sapphires. 3 *c.* 1945–49. Polished-copper bangle, raised-stud design to front, hinge and clip side fastening. 4 *c.* 1940. Wide polished-brass bangle, painted design of butterflies and flowers, brass edges, open back. 5 *c.* 1949. Polished-copper bangle, contemporary design, hinged back, open front. 6 *c.* 1948. Wide matt-silver bangle, design of raised studs and twisted wire, open back. 7 *c.* 1945. Carved clear yellow plastic bangle, inset design of mushrooms. 8 *c.* 1945–49. Painted plastic bangle, oriental heads complete with fake gem-set crowns, collars and earrings, elasticated joints. 9 *c.* 1941–45. Bracelet of imitation-turquoise flowers, coloured bead centres with pierced gilded ribbon loops, matching chain and fixings. In the style of Miriam Haskell. 10 *c.* 1948. Gold bracelet, strap and buckle design. 11 *c.* 1949. Platinum bracelet, foliate-design rectangular plaques set with brilliant-cut diamonds. 12 *c.* 1940. Linked floral-design polished-brass bracelet, two-colour enamel. 13 *c.* 1940. Polished-brass bracelet, linked plaques, pressed floral design, touched with coloured enamels. 14 *c.* 1945–49. Platinum bracelet, central panel set with cushion-shaped sapphires, brilliant-cut diamonds set between, matching articulated bracelet back. In the style of Cartier. 15 *c.* 1949. Gold-coloured metal bracelet composed of engraved rectangular plaques and domed polished coloured glass, gold bead spacers.

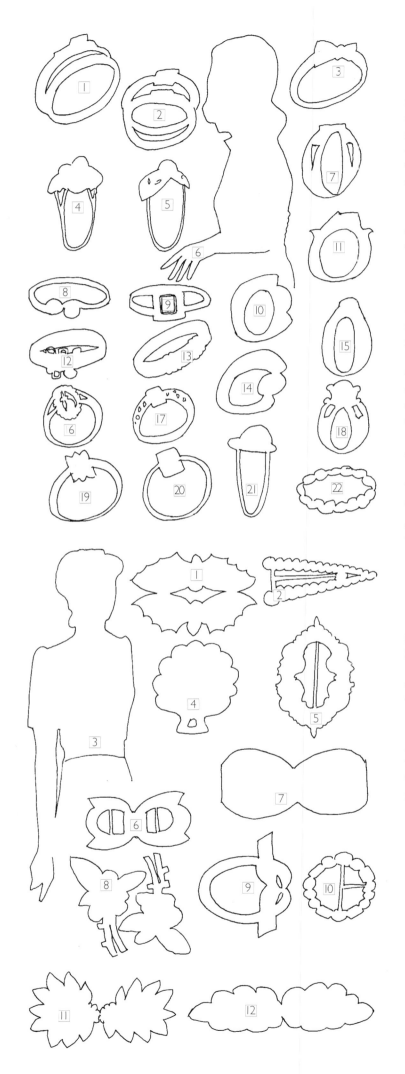

Rings 1940–1949

1 c. 948. Matching gold wedding and engagement rings set with pale sapphires. 2 c. 1948. Matching gold wedding and engagement rings set with pale rubies. 3 c. 1945. Gold ring, wide band, looped design set with diamonds. 4 c. 1949. Platinum ring, foliate design set with diamonds and emeralds. 5 c. 1949. Bronze ring, foliate design, set with coloured-glass stones. 6 c. 1948. Matching gold wedding and engagement rings set with diamonds. 7 c. 1940–45. Gold ring, wide band, architectural design set with onyx and diamonds, open shoulders. 8 c. 1940. Gold engagement ring, two large diamonds set between cross-over shoulders. 9 c. 1945. Gold ring, cushion-shaped diamond claw set within a rectangular surround, baguette-cut diamond shoulders. 10 c. 1940–45. Gold ring, wide band, architectural design, domed central pane set with diamonds, shoulders set with rubies and sapphires. 11 c. 1940–45. Gold ring, architectural design, central roof-shaped panel set with diamonds. 12 c. 1945. Gold ring, wide band, asymmetric design set with single ruby and diamonds. 13 c. 1945. Gold ring, wide band, single diamond set between raised bars. 14 c. 1949. Gold ring, rigid band, diamonds set between platinum trim. 15 c. 1940–45. Silver ring, wide band, set with cabochon stone. 16 c. 1940. Silver ring, pierced design set with marcasites. 17 c. 1940–45. Silver ring set with cushion-shaped stone, pierced shoulders. 18 c. 1940–45. Gold ring, wide band, crown design set with diamonds and emeralds. 19 c. 1940. Platinum ring, pierced oblong plaque set with two large diamonds, surround of smaller diamonds. 20 c. 1940. Silver ring, cushion-shaped stone with marcasite surround. 21 c. 1949. Gold ring, large cabochon turquoise surround of marcasites and fake diamonds. 22 c. 1949. Silver eternity ring, linked heart-shaped design set with coloured stones.

Buckles and Clasps 1940–1949

1 c. 1940–45. Polished and etched brass buckle, moth design. 2 c. 1940–45. Arrowhead-shaped brass buckle, set with multicoloured glass stones, single prong. 3 c. 1945. Oval plastic clasp, openwork geometric design. 4 c. 1945. Cast brass buckle peacock design, multicoloured enamel decoration. 5 c. 1940–49. Gilded-metal buckle, delicate openwork design set with coloured-glass stones. 6 c. 1945. Carved Bakelite clasp, cut-out D-shaped centres 7 c. 1940–45. Moulded frosted-glass clasp, geometric design, scalloped edges. 8 c. 1945–49. Silver-washed-metal clasp, pair of matching flowers, set with white and coloured paste stones. 9 c. 1948. Oval metal buckle, tied ribbon design, enamelled in two colours, set with cabochon fake-turquoise stones. 10 c. 1940. Small round gold-washed-brass buckle, set with moulded coloured-glass stones. 11 c. 1945. Gold-washed-plastic clasp, foliate design, floral clasps set with coloured-glass stones. 12 c. 1945. Carved marbled-Bakelite clasp, facing stylized leaf design.

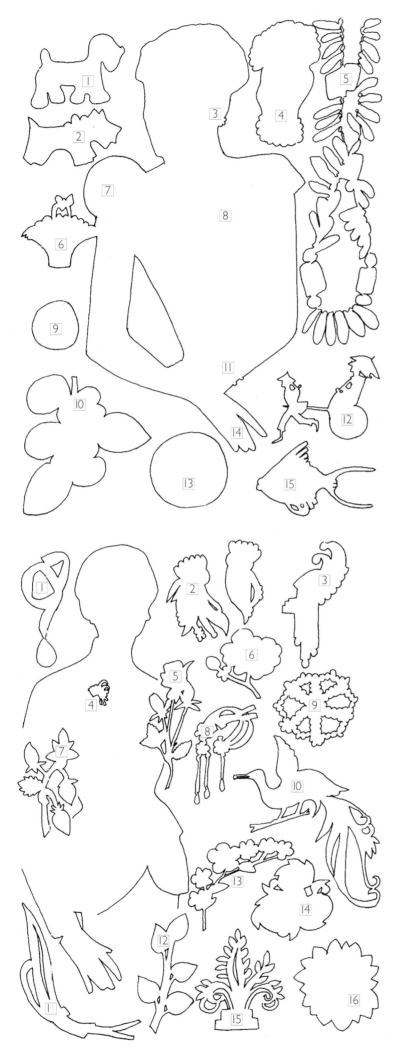

Novelty Jewelry 1940–1949

1 *c.* 1940. Polished-brass brooch, cartoon-dog design with engraved features. 2 *c.* 1945. Pressed-plastic brooch, scottie-dog design, painted fur, eye, tongue and ribbon-bow collar. 3 *c.* 1945–49. Plastic clip-on earrings, multicoloured fruit and basket design. 4 *c.* 1945. Polished pressed-metal clip, Carmen Miranda head decorated with fruit and flowers. 5 *c.* 1945. Short necklace, comprising tiny plastic bananas spaced by various sized plastic or wooden beads and marbled-plastic plaques. 6 *c.* 1945. Pressed-metal brooch, multicoloured painted flowers arranged in gold painted basket. 7 *c.* 1940–45. Round brooch decorated with multicoloured wooden beads and buttons. 8 *c.* 1949. Painted wood necklace, with fringe of hand-shaped leaves suspended from handcarved wooden beads. 9 *c.* 1945–49. Round transparent-plastic brooch, inset lady in crinoline holding parasol and standing among flowers, all in pastel colours. 10 *c.* 1945–49. Dyed stockinette corsage brooch, composed of finely wired leaf shapes, bound in green or gold, with pink and white plastic stamen centres. 11 *c.* 1949. White plastic-bead bracelet, matching cluster of yellow-centred flowers set among leaves at front. 12 *c.* 1949. Polished-brass brooch, design of coolie pulling rickshaw with passenger, set with coloured stones. 13 *c.* 1945–49. Round ceramic hand-modelled brooch mounted on a brass back plate, design of raised hand-painted flowers within a gold painted border. 14 *c.* 1940. Plastic ring with rectangular panel displaying a miniature photograph. 15 *c.* 1945. Stylized fish brooch, polished-brass finish, set with coloured-glass stones.

Brooches and Clips 1950–1953

1 *c.* 1950. Silver-coloured metal brooch, twisted-ribbon design, pavé-set clear paste stones, matching pear-shaped pendant. 2 *c.* 1950. Two non-matching dress clips, foliate design, white gold set with diamonds and sapphires. 3 *c.* 1950. Cascade brooch, pavé-set brilliant- and baguette-cut diamonds. 4 *c.* 1950. Fan-shaped gold-coloured metal lapel clip, finished with ribbon loops and ends set with clear paste stones. 5 *c.* 1952. Enamelled metal brooch, rose-spray design, highlighted with rows of marcasites. 6 *c.* 1950–53. Multi-gem-set gold brooch, flowerhead design, central cabochon ruby within border of brilliant-cut diamonds, outer surround of cabochon sapphires, emeralds and rubies. In the style of Boucheron. 7 *c.* 1953. Gilded-metal brooch, stylized fruit and flower spray, set with clear and coloured paste stones. 8 *c.* 1953. Silver brooch, set with white zircons, matching pear-shaped drops under line of synthetic white sapphire baguettes. 9 *c.* 1952. Wired glass-bead brooch. 10 *c.* 1953. Silver-coloured metal brooch, bird design, details touched with coloured enamels and set with small rhinestones. 11 *c.* 1950–53. Foliate-design brooch, set with clear and coloured-glass stones. 12 *c.* 1953. Foliate-design gilded-metal dress clip, painted stem, leaves set with rhinestones. 13 *c.* 1953. Gold spray brooch, pearl flower centres, synthetic cabochon ruby surround, leaves set with matching synthetic emeralds. 14 *c.* 1950. Dress clip, set with green crystals among gold-coloured metal leaves. 15 *c.* 1953. Tree brooch set with rhinestones and decorated with multicoloured glass leaves. 16 *c.* 1952. Flowerhead brooch, wired plastic-coral and silver-metal bead petals, rhinestone stamens.

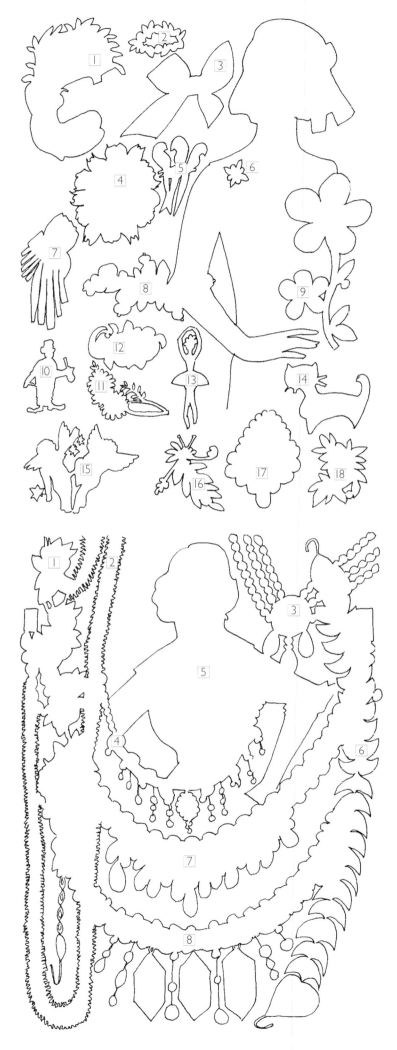

Brooches and Clips 1954–1959

1 *c.* 1955. Large gilt-bronze tree brooch, silver nymph sitting at base, matching bird on branch. In the style of Line Vautrin. 2 *c.* 1959. Oval brooch with open centre, foliate design set with multicoloured moulded-glass stones. 3 *c.* 1955. Gold ribbon brooch, pavé-set with brilliant-cut diamonds edged with calibre-cut emeralds. 4 *c.* 1958. Round metal brooch, central iridescent glass stone, matching smaller stones in decorative borders. 5 *c.* 1959. Gilded-metal brooch, three birds on a branch, fake-pearl bodies, rhinestone eyes, matching stones in long tail feathers. 6 *c.* 1959. Gilded-silver brooch, set with coloured-glass cabochon stones and rhinestones. 7 *c.* 1955. Gold brooch set with brilliant-cut diamonds, looped spray set with baguette stones. 8 *c.* 1955. Gilded-metal branch-shaped brooch, imitation pearl and diamond flower heads set among seed-pearl leaves. In the style of Miriam Haskell. 9 *c.* 1959. Large gilded-metal floral spray brooch, prong-set moulded coloured-glass petals and leaves, clear glass centres, matching curved stem. 10 *c.* 1959. Gold clown holding violin, set with sapphires, rubies and diamonds. 11 *c.* 1955–59. Floral spray brooch, pale aquamarine and diamond flowers among gold leaves and stems. 12 *c.* 1955. Two clips of individual design forming an openwork silver brooch set with tiny rhinestones. 13 *c.* 1955. Gold ballerina brooch, pearl head with diamond tiara, matching bracelets, dress and shoes. 14 *c* 1955–59. Gold-coloured metal cat brooch, plastic head and body. 15 *c* 1955. Gold-washed cherubs set with rhinestones. In the style of Corc. 16 *c.* 1959. Gilded-metal foliate-spray brooch, set with moulded coloured-glass stones. 17 *c.* 1959. Waterfall brooch, plastic beads in graded sizes and shaded colours wired onto a gilded-plastic disc. 18 *c.* 1959. Floral spray brooch set with moulded two-colour iridescent glass stones.

Necklaces 1950–1954

1 *c.* 1950. Short plastic necklace, composed of flat leaf-shaped plates decorated with two three-dimensional flowers in contrasting colours, each flower with clear glass stone centre, the plates connected with gold-coloured metal chain, matching fastenings. 2 *c.* 1950–54. Long imitation coral necklace, no fastenings. 3 *c.* 1952–54. Three-strand graded imitation pearl necklace, large central plaque set with rhinestones and seed pearls, finished with three large pear-shaped droplets. 4 *c.* 1952–54. Short necklace, tapered baguette-cut diamond front section with brilliant-cut diamond drops suspended from loops of pavé-set diamond scrolls, large pear-shaped diamond centre stone, diamond-set back chain. 5 *c.* 1954. Three-strand plastic-bead necklace, various sized beads in two colours. 6 *c.* 1954. Gilded finely textured bronze necklace, flexible design based on the vertebrae, heart-shaped end plaques with hook fastenings. In the style of Line Vautrin. 7 *c.* 1952–54. Short choker necklace, two rows of equal-sized imitation pearls, spaced by small coloured-glass beads and white paste stones, pear-shaped pearls in groups of three suspended on fine chain under central section, rhinestone-set fastening. 8 *c.* 1954. Multicoloured glass and plastic bead necklace, three rows of various sized beads, matching pendant beads and three large moulded-plastic drops.

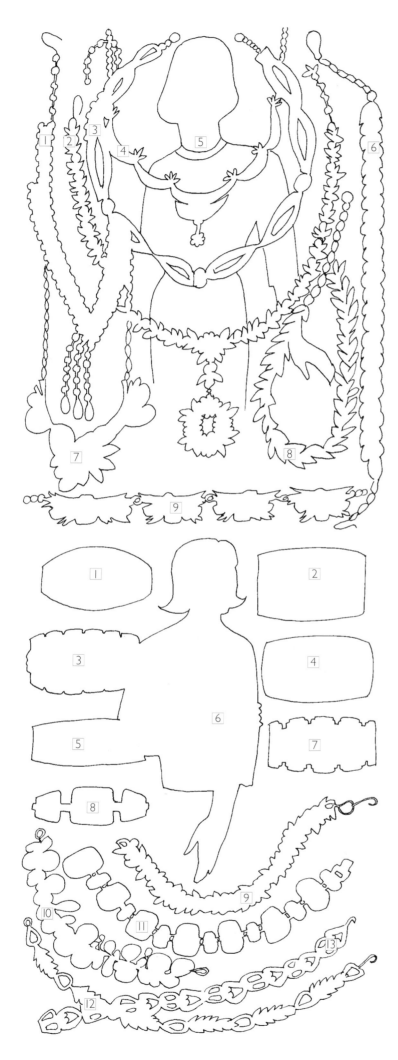

Necklaces 1955–1959

1 c. 1958. Asymmetric-design necklace, composed of one, two and three strands of multicoloured faceted glass stones linked by flat-silver strips, ending with three-strand pendant with peardrop fake-pearl tips. 2 c. 1959. Transparent multicoloured glass stone foliate-design necklace, matching central pendant wreath, hook fastening. 3 c. 1955. Silver-plated metal necklace, twisted-rope design, set with various sized faceted rhinestones, matching disc spacers, chain back. 4 c. 1955. Diamond and platinum necklace composed of baguette-cut diamond swags with brilliant-cut diamond swags below, matching central pendant section, single row of diamonds to back fastening. 5 c. 1958. Gold choker necklace, brick-link design, bead edging to top and bottom. 6 c. 1959. Gold-plated silver choker necklace, foliate design, set with fake cabochon emerald and sapphire beads, matching smaller faceted stones on outer edge, chain-link back. 7 c. 1958. Asymmetric gold-plated pendant necklace, composed of various sized pear-shaped polished semi-precious stones, set within scrollwork design, offset by faceted coloured stones in fancy settings, chain back. 8 c. 1958. Gold-coloured metal necklace, composed of curved branch shapes set with multicoloured enamelled leaves, chain back. 9 c. 1959. Engraved matt-silver necklace, composed of foliate-design plaques set with random-shaped multicoloured semi-precious stones, chain back.

Bracelets and Bangles 1950–1959

1 c. 1955–59. Polished beaten-copper bangle, engraved design of cats within painted background. 2 c. 1959. Wide gilded-metal bangle, raised design of deer against textured background. 3 c. 1950. Polished-silver linked bracelet, composed of shaped plaques decorated with gold-washed cameo-style classical heads, narrow spacing plaques set with panels of fake jade. 4 c. 1952. Wide gilded-metal bangle, decorated with coral beads and gold wire. In the style of Miriam Haskell. 5 c. 1950. Linked bracelet, interlocking shaped plaques set with brilliant-cut diamonds. 6 c. 1950. Wide metal bangle, multicoloured enamel and gold design against white background. 7 c. 1950. Linked bracelet, pierced plaques set with brilliant-cut diamonds surrounding pavé-set central panels, matching solid hinged links. 8 c. 1955. Gold-plated bracelet composed of multicoloured enamelled plaques of geometric design, narrow links. 9 c. 1953–55. Fine silver bracelet, composed of interlocking foliate-design motifs, set with coloured-glass stones and fake pearls, leaves painted with coloured enamels. 10 c. 1955–59. Multicoloured glass-bead charm-style bracelet, gold-coloured metal wire links and fastenings. 11 c. 1959. Gold-coloured metal linked bracelet, composed of irregular-shaped enamelled plaques, matching smaller spacing plaques. 12 c. 1955. Silver bracelet, composed of moulded pink glass leaves and alternating rhinestone-set links. 13 c. 1953. Linked bracelet set with imitation diamonds, gilded-silver links and fastenings.

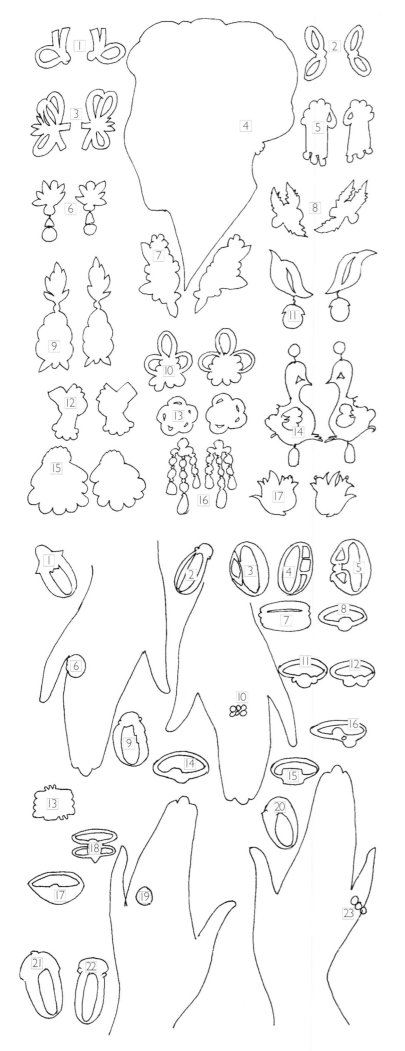

Earrings 1950–1959

1 c. 1953. Silver clip-on earrings, loop-and-tail design, set with diamonds. 2 c. 1953. Gold clip-on earrings, loop design set with diamonds. 3 c. 1953. Silver clip-on earrings, double loop-and-tail design, set with diamonds. 4 c. 1958. Clip-on earrings, round metal plate decorated with plastic beads. 5 c. 1950–55. Diamond clip-on earrings, spray-and-scroll design with sapphire highlights, matching detachable triple row of baguette-cut diamond drops. 6 c. 1955. Diamond earrings, foliate design, detachable pendants. 7 c. 1959. Large clip-on earrings, spray of plastic flowers glued onto transparent plate. 8 c. 1959. Clip-on gold painted metal earrings, three multicoloured glass stones arranged with painted leaves. 9 c. 1955. Long pendant earrings, pear-shaped coloured paste stone set within wreath of clear stones, matching clips. 10 c. 1958. Pale multicoloured heart-shaped glass stones against loops set with small clear glass stones. 11 c. 1958. Engraved and painted leaf-shaped metal clip-on earrings, matching caps above fake-pearl drops. 12 c. 1950–55. Small diamond clip-on earrings, pierced hoop and scroll design. 13 c. 1959. Clip-on gilt earrings, knot design set with fake-turquoise stones, large central fake pearl. 14 c. 1955. Gilt pendant earrings, fish design, set with fake pearls, matching clips and pear-shaped drops. 15 c. 1955–59. Clip-on earrings, transparent plastic plate decorated with clear plastic stones and two rows of plastic pearl drops to one side. 16 c. 1955. Pendant earrings, moulded plastic beads spaced with gold metal beads and ending in pear-shaped drops. 17 c. 1959. Clip-on earrings, floral design enamelled in multicolours.

Rings 1950–1959

1 c. 1950–55. Gold ring, domed turquoise stone in fancy setting spaced with diamonds. 2 c. 1955. Two hoop gold ring, set with cabochon ruby. 3 c. 1955. Two hoop gold ring, joined at back, set with coloured stone. 4 c. 1955. Two hoop ring, joined at back, set with large emerald and two diamonds. 5 c. 1955–59. Yellow gold ring, open shoulders, central sapphire set in white gold. 6 c. 1955–59. Layered-petal-design gold ring, central cabochon stone. 7 c. 1950–55. Wide gold band, central rib, spotted with diamonds. 8 c. 1955. Gold ring, solitaire diamond, diamond-set shoulders. 9 c. 1958. Gold ring, single cabochon stone, stepped shoulders. 10 c. 1959. Crossover diamond-set ring, ruby stops. 11 c. 1955. Gold ring, solitaire diamond, decorative diamond-set shoulders. 12 c. 1955. Gold ring, two closely set brilliant-cut diamonds, diamond-set shoulders. 13 c. 1959. Wide ribbed gold band, surmounted with diamonds and rubies. 14 c. 1959. Two brilliant-cut diamonds set at an angle to each other, diamond-set shoulders. 15 c. 1950. Gold ring, set with sapphires and diamonds. 16 c. 1955–59. Gold crossover ring set with diamonds. 17 c. 1959. Gold ring, shaped front set with cabochon emerald against background of diamonds. 18 c. 1955. Pear-shaped diamond set between two gold bands. 19 c. 1955–59. Ring composed of a fake-pearl surrounded by rows of glass beads. 20 c. 1955–59. Silver ring, domed front and shoulders set with rhinestones and edged with fake emeralds. 21 c. 1959. Gold ring set with emeralds and diamonds against a diamond-set background. 22 c. 1959. Wide copper ring, semi-precious stone set in silver wire. 23 c. 1950. Gold ring set with three fake pearls.

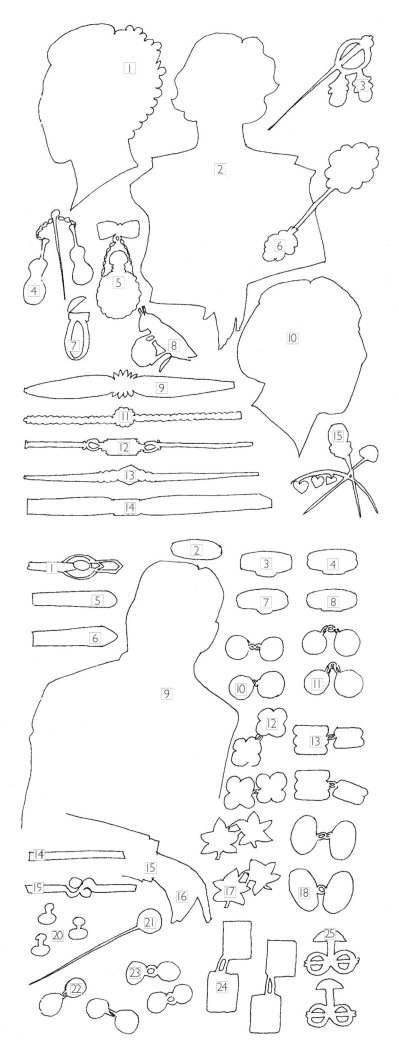

Miscellaneous Jewelry and Jewelled Pieces 1940–1959

1 *c.* 1948–50. Asymmetric hair decoration, multicoloured wired blown-glass grapes set among stamped velvet leaves. 2 *c.* 1948–50. Wide silk-organdie collar, embroidered with glass beads in a design of leaves and berries. 3 *c.* 1949. Gilded-silver lapel pin, set with rhinestones and coloured-glass stones, matching pendant drops. 4 *c.* 1940–42. Gold lapel pin, miniature mandolin and violin suspended from fine chain. 5 *c.* 1940–42. Gilded bow knot brooch set with tiny rhinestones, matching perfume bottle suspended from fine chain. 6 *c.* 1955–59. Large gilt lapel pin, set with large multicoloured cut-glass stones in floral arrangement, matching endstop. 7 *c.* 1948. Gold ring, miniature watch concealed under hinged jewelled lid. 8 *c.* 1940–45. Brooch watch, grasshopper design set with diamonds, coloured enamel details, matching watch case. 9 *c.* 1959. Gold wristwatch, sunburst design, woven gold mesh strap. 10 *c.* 1958–59. Hair bandeau, flower-and-leaf design covered with multicoloured glass beads and spaced with rhinestones. In the style of Miriam Haskell. 11 *c.* 1950–55. Wristwatch, mother-of-pearl face set in round case, diamond surround, matching narrow strap. 12 *c.* 1945–50. Wristwatch, oblong case set with diamonds in a geometric stepped design, fine silk cord strap. 13 *c.* 1945–50. Wristwatch, rectangular case set with diamonds and small rubies, matching shoulders, silk cord strap. 14 *c.* 1940–45. Wristwatch, dark face set in plain gold rectangular case, wide strap in two-gold brick-link design. 15 *c.* 1951. Three hatpins: curved gold pin with pendant polished ruby hearts; silver pin, black plastic spotted with rhinestones, matching base; gilt pin, domed plastic head with painted spots.

Men's Jewelry 1940–1959

1 *c.* 1945–55. Chromium-plated tie clip, enamelled pattern on central lozenge. 2 *c.* 1955–59. Gold ring with claw-set rectangular ruby. 3 *c.* 1950–55. Gold signet ring, plain face, raised shoulders. 4 *c.* 1950–55. Ribbed gold ring, plain face with engraved edges. 5 *c.* 1950–55. Polished-copper tie clip. 6 *c.* 1955–59. Gold tie clip set with synthetic cabochon sapphire on pointed edge. 7 *c.* 1955–59. Gold ring set with cabochon emerald, raised shoulders. 8 *c.* 1955–59. Gold signet ring, rectangular face set with tiny diamonds in two corners. 9 *c.* 1959. Gold tie clip set with rectangular ruby. 10 *c.* 1940–45. Gold-plated balls decorated with circular synthetic sapphires in fancy settings, chain links. 11 *c.* 1950–55. Gold-plated fluted balls, set with single cabochon rubies on bases, chain links. 12 *c.* 1955. Quatrefoil opaque stone cufflinks, gold ropework ties, chain links. 13 *c.* 1940–45. Cufflinks composed of coral batons bound with gold ropework, chain links. 14 *c.* 1950–59. Gold tie pin, set with single pearl. 15 *c.* 1959. Gold cufflinks, leaf design set with cabochon ruby. 16 *c.* 1959. Gold ring set with small diamond in centre of plain face. 17 *c.* 1950–59. Gold cufflinks, ivy-leaf design set with calibré-cut emeralds, clip connections. 18 *c.* 1945–49. Textured-gold oval cufflinks, chain links. 19 *c.* 1959. Gold tie pin, twisted design set with two pearls. 20 *c.* 1959. Three gold dress studs, set with single pearls. 21 *c.* 1955. Gold stickpin, large pearl head. 22 *c.* 1955–59. Gold cufflinks set with half pearls. 23 *c.* 1950–55. Pale sapphire cufflinks with diamond collet centres, clip connections. 24 *c.* 1945–49. Platinum cufflinks, front plates set with sapphires and diamonds, engraved back plates, single clip connections. 25 *c.* 1955. Polished twisted copper-wire cufflinks, rod and bar connections.

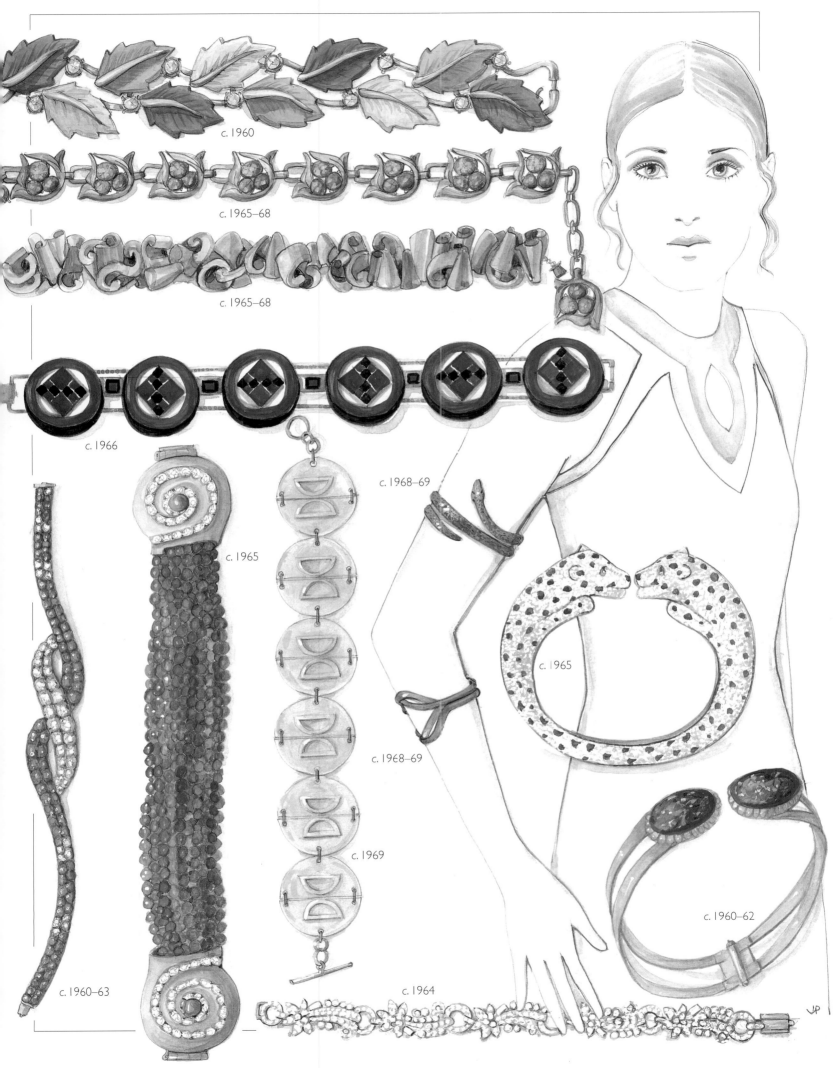

c. 1960

c. 1965–68

c. 1965–68

c. 1966

c. 1965

c. 1968–69

c. 1960–63

c. 1968–69

c. 1969

c. 1965

c. 1964

c. 1960–62

Brooches 1960–1969

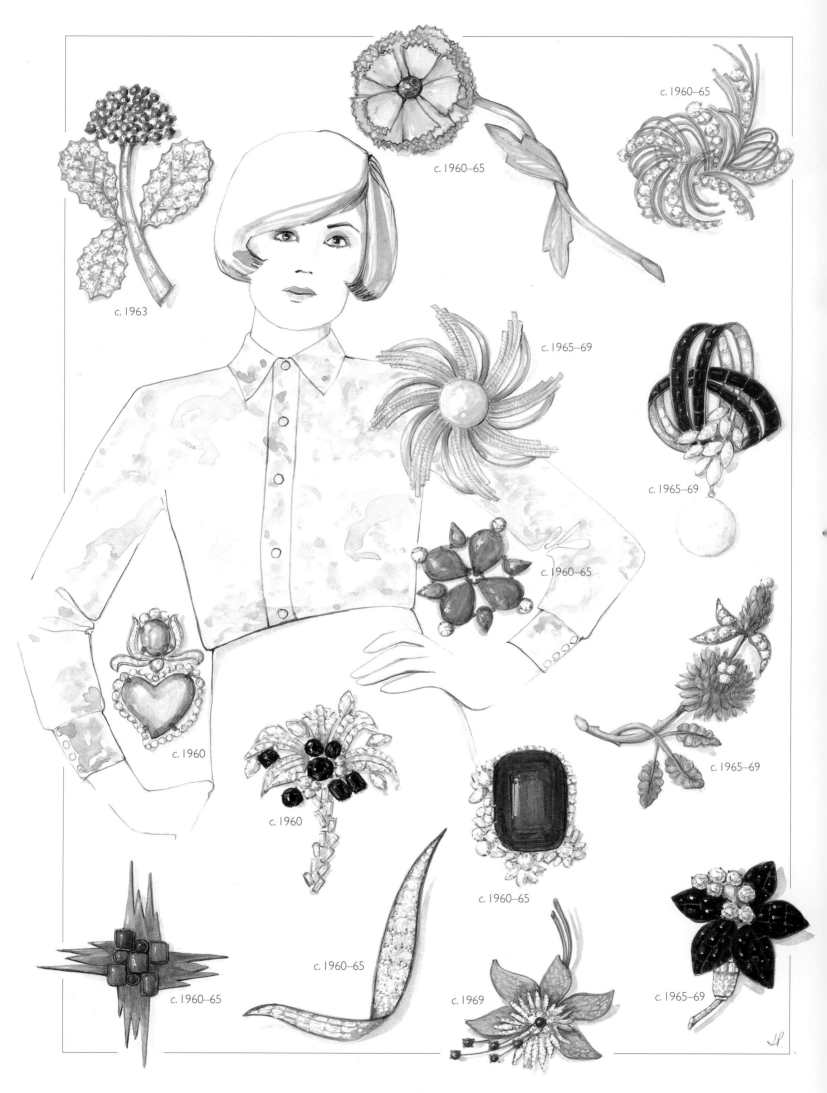

c. 1960–65

c. 1960–65

c. 1963

c. 1965–69

c. 1965–69

c. 1965–69

c. 1960–65

c. 1960

c. 1965–69

c. 1960

c. 1960–65

c. 1960–65

c. 1960–65

c. 1969

c. 1965–69

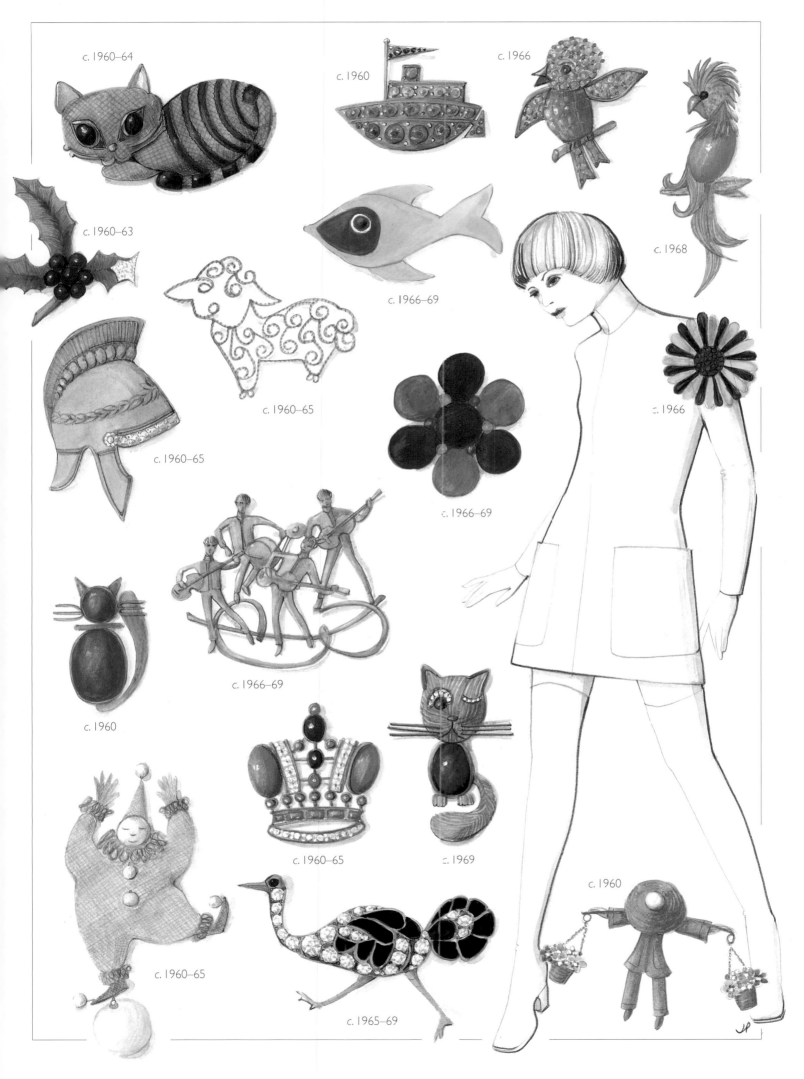

c. 1960–64

c. 1960

c. 1966

c. 1968

c. 1960–63

c. 1966–69

c. 1966

c. 1960–65

c. 1960–65

c. 1966–69

c. 1960

c. 1966–69

c. 1960

c. 1960–65

c. 1969

c. 1960

c. 1960–65

c. 1965–69

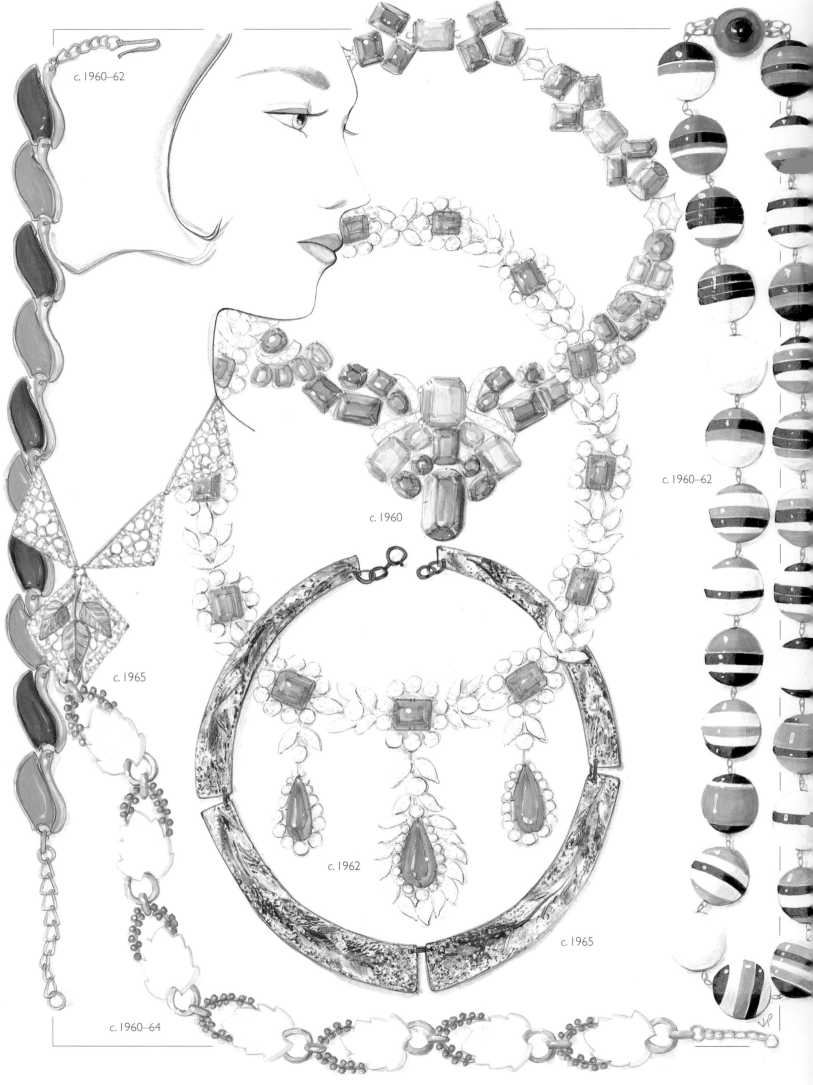

c. 1960–62

c. 1960

c. 1960–62

c. 1965

c. 1962

c. 1965

c. 1960–64

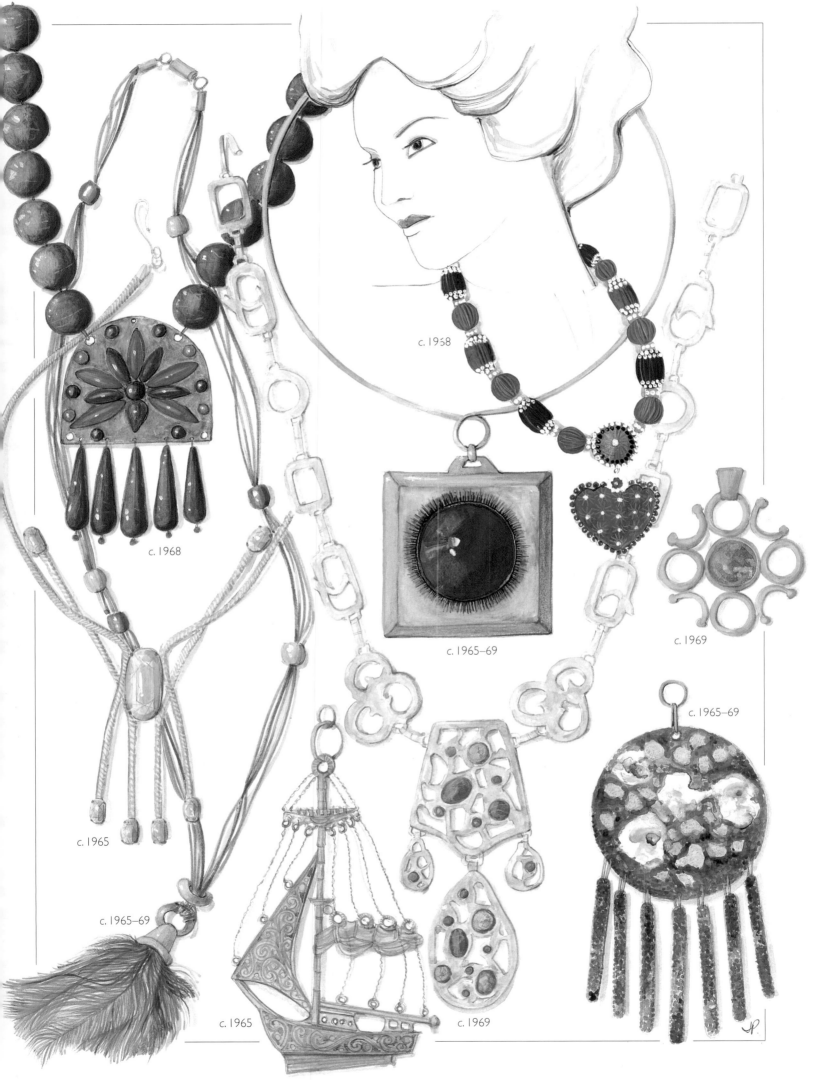

c.1968

c.1965

c.1965–69

c.1965

c.1958

c.1965–69

c.1969

c.1969

c.1965–69

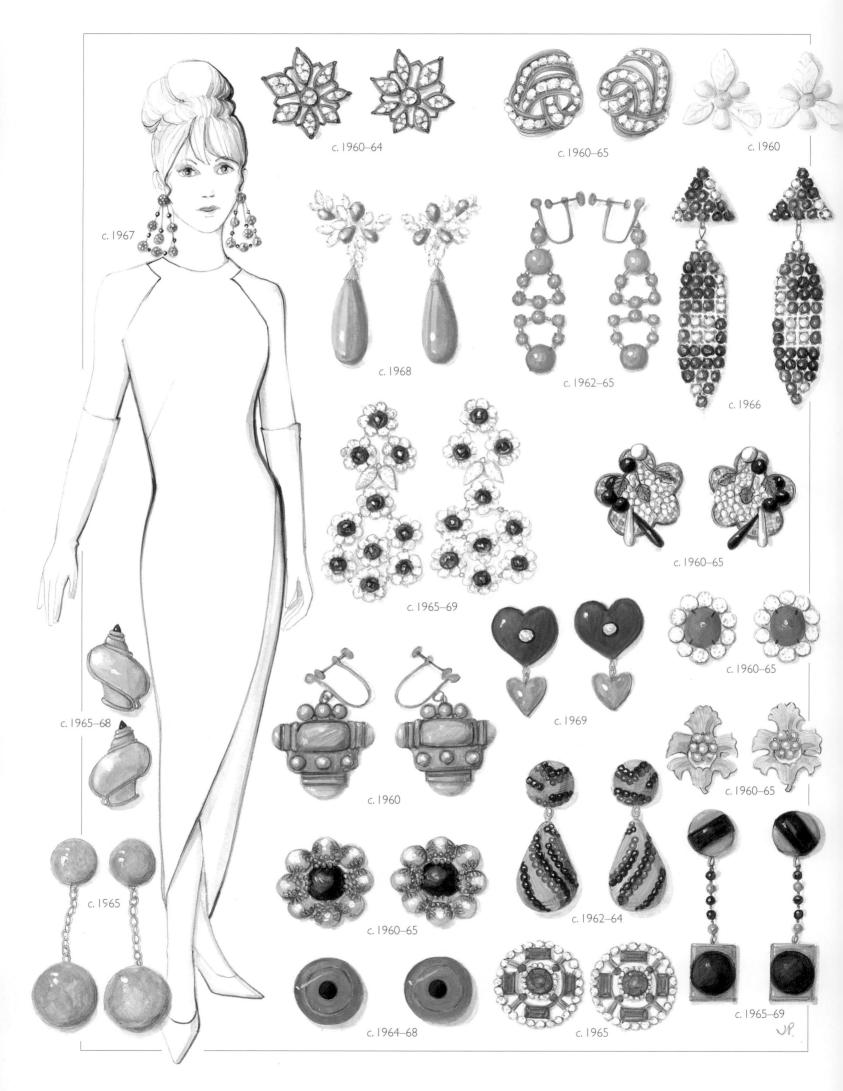

Earrings 1960–1969

c. 1960–64

c. 1960–65

c. 1960

c. 1967

c. 1968

c. 1962–65

c. 1966

c. 1965–69

c. 1960–65

c. 1965–68

c. 1969

c. 1960–65

c. 1960

c. 1960–65

c. 1965

c. 1960–65

c. 1962–64

c. 1964–68

c. 1965

c. 1965–69

JP.

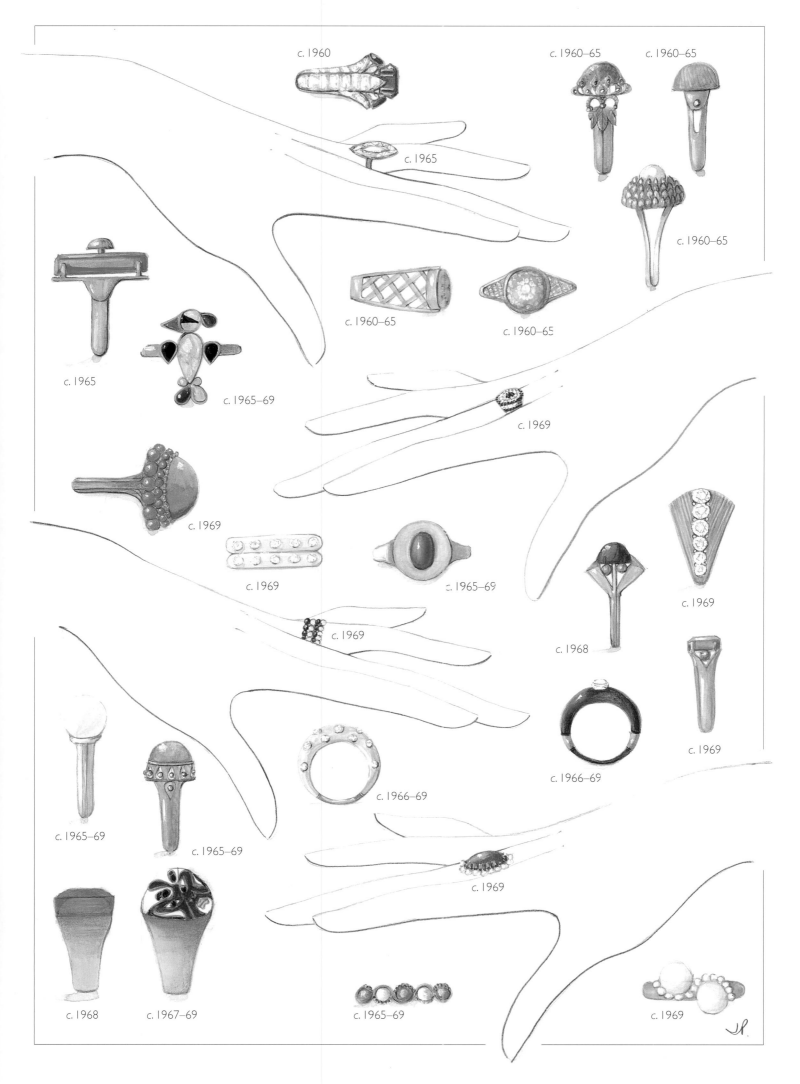

c. 1960

c. 1965

c. 1960–65

c. 1960–65

c. 1960–65

c. 1965

c. 1960–65

c. 1960–65

c. 1965–69

c. 1969

c. 1969

c. 1969

c. 1969

c. 1965–69

c. 1968

c. 1969

c. 1969

c. 1966–69

c. 1965–69

c. 1965–69

c. 1966–69

c. 1969

c. 1968

c. 1967–69

c. 1965–69

c. 1969

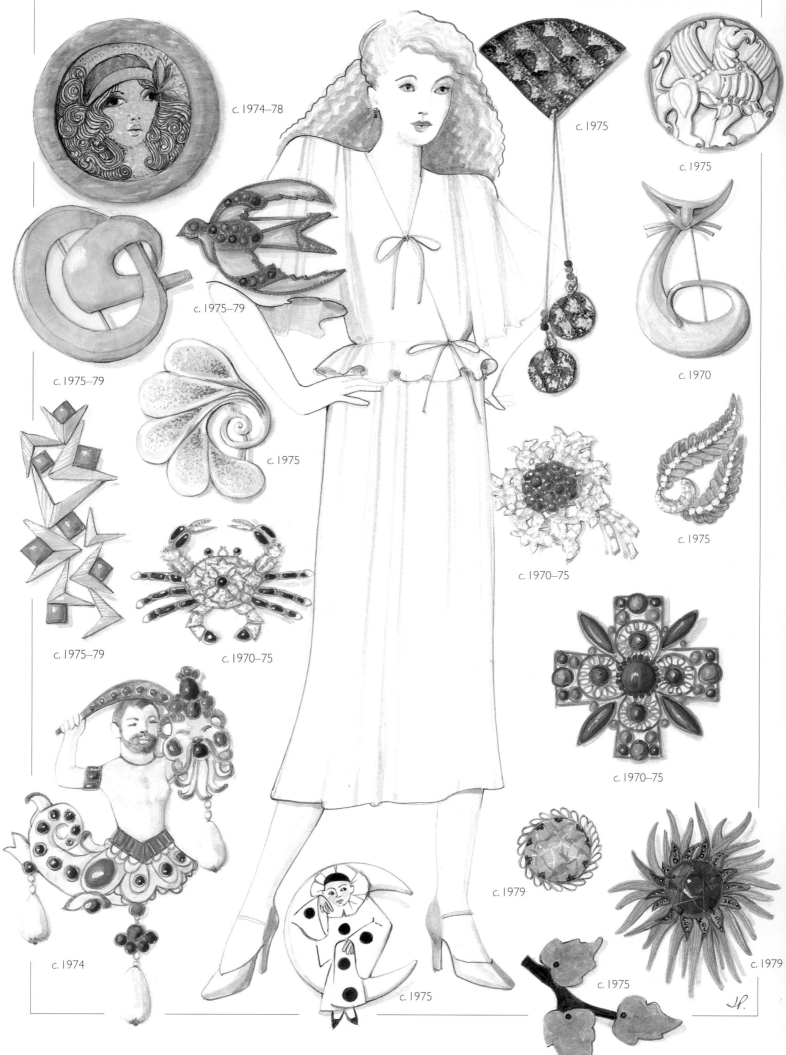

c. 1974–78

c. 1975

c. 1975

c. 1975

c. 1975–79

c. 1970

c. 1975–79

c. 1975

c. 1975

c. 1970–75

c. 1975–79

c. 1970–75

c. 1970–75

c. 1974

c. 1979

c. 1975

c. 1975

c. 1979

88

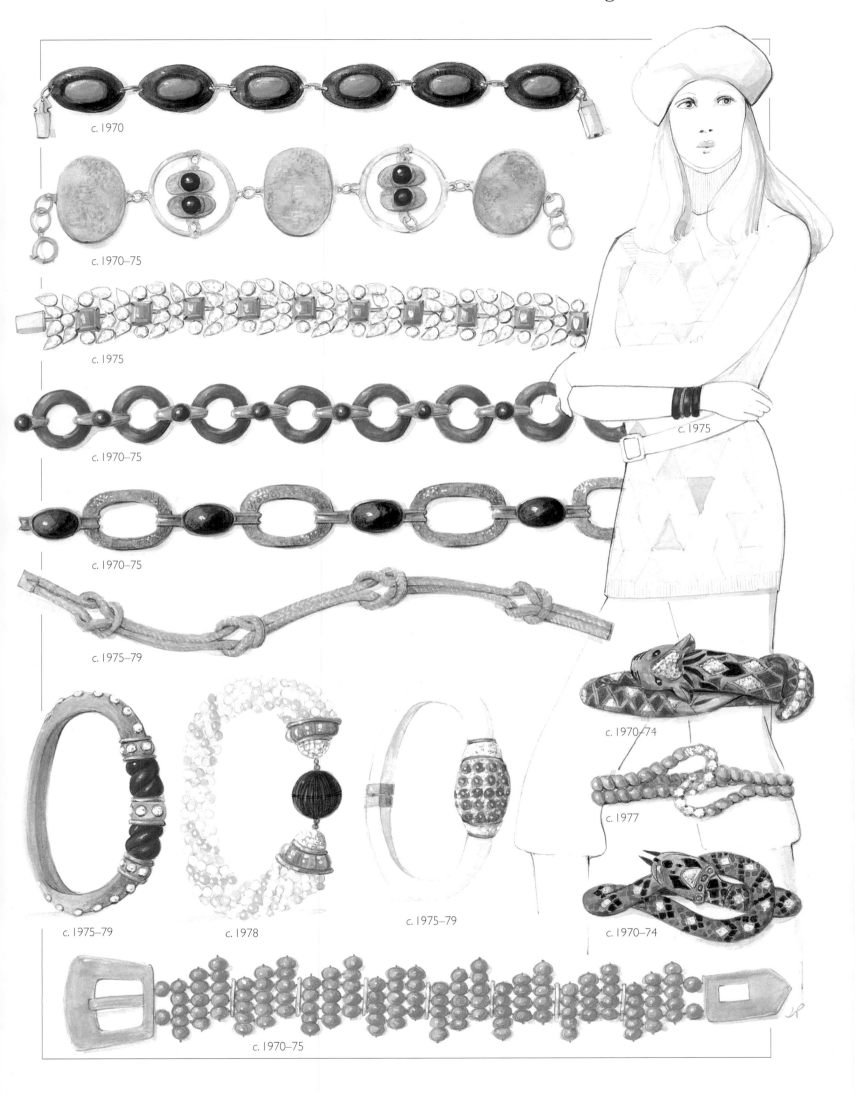

c. 1970

c. 1970–75

c. 1975

c. 1970–75

c. 1970–75

c. 1975–79

c. 1975

c. 1975–79

c. 1978

c. 1975–79

c. 1970–74

c. 1977

c. 1970–74

c. 1970–75

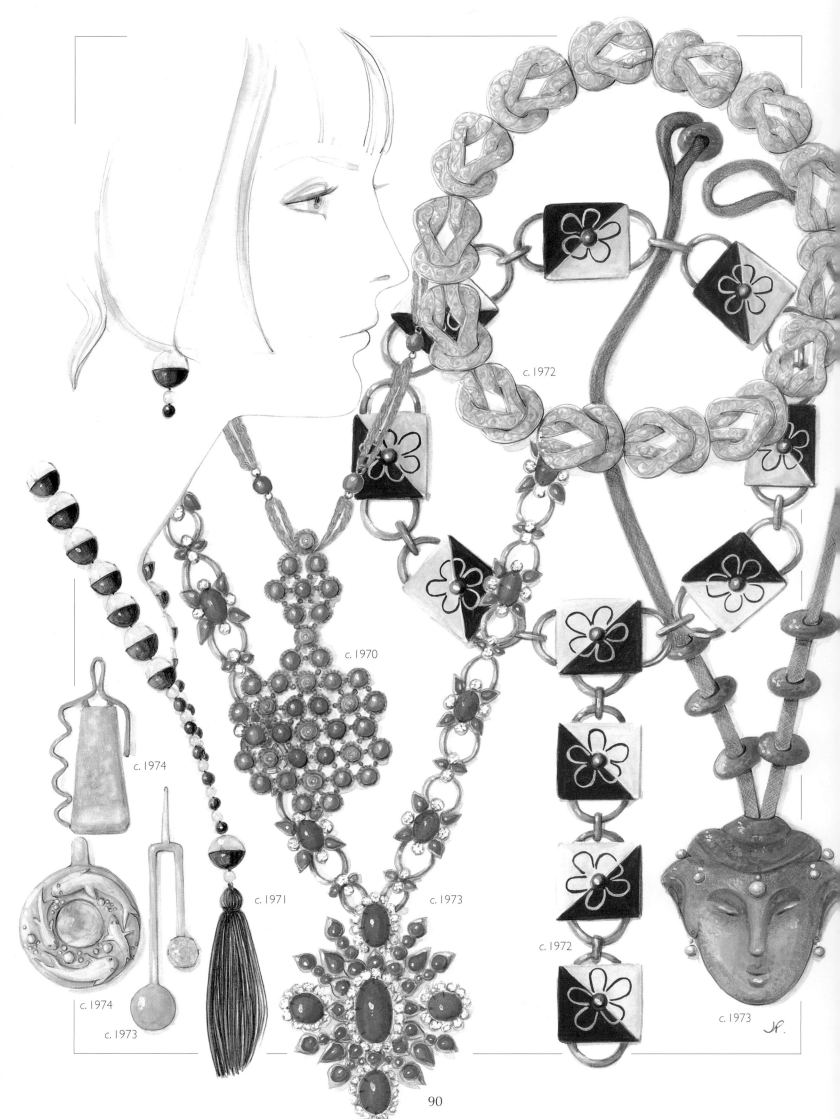

c. 1972

c. 1970

c. 1974

c. 1971

c. 1973

c. 1972

c. 1974

c. 1973

c. 1973

c. 1972

c. 1973

JP.

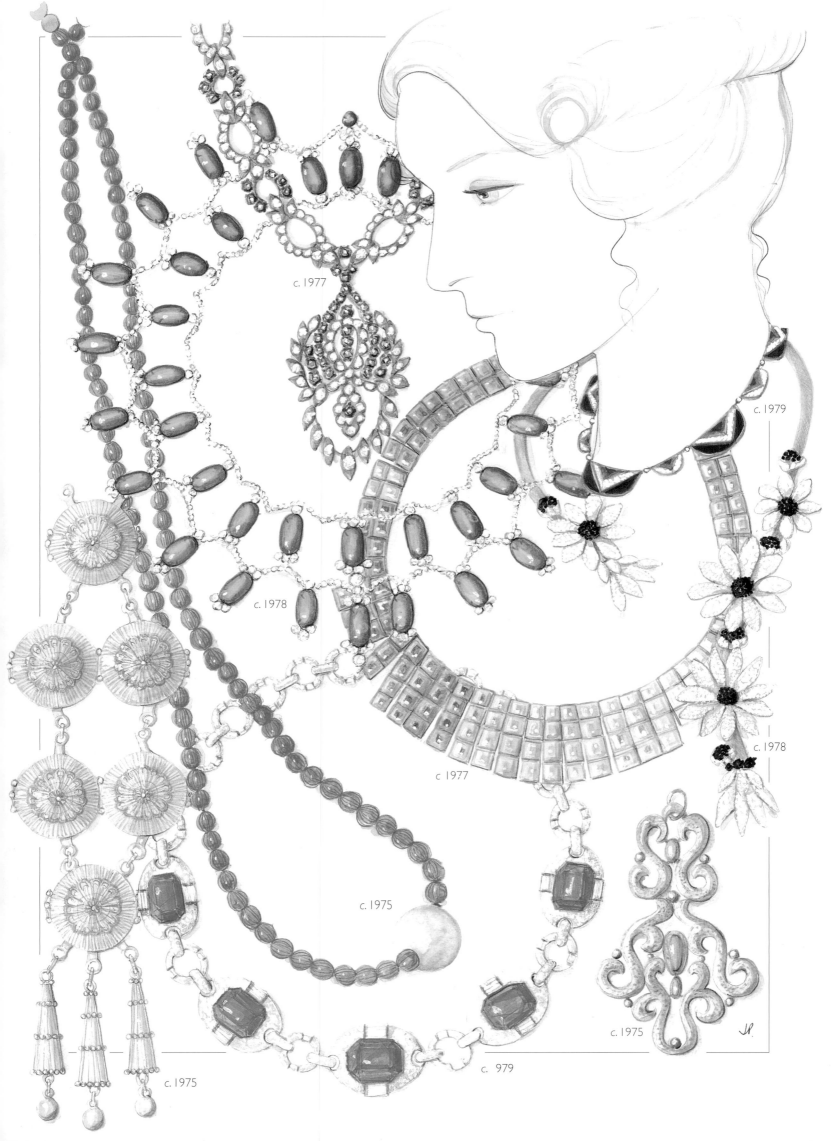

c. 1977

c. 1979

c. 1978

c. 1977

c. 1978

c. 1975

c. 1975

c. 1975

c. 1975

c. 979

JP.

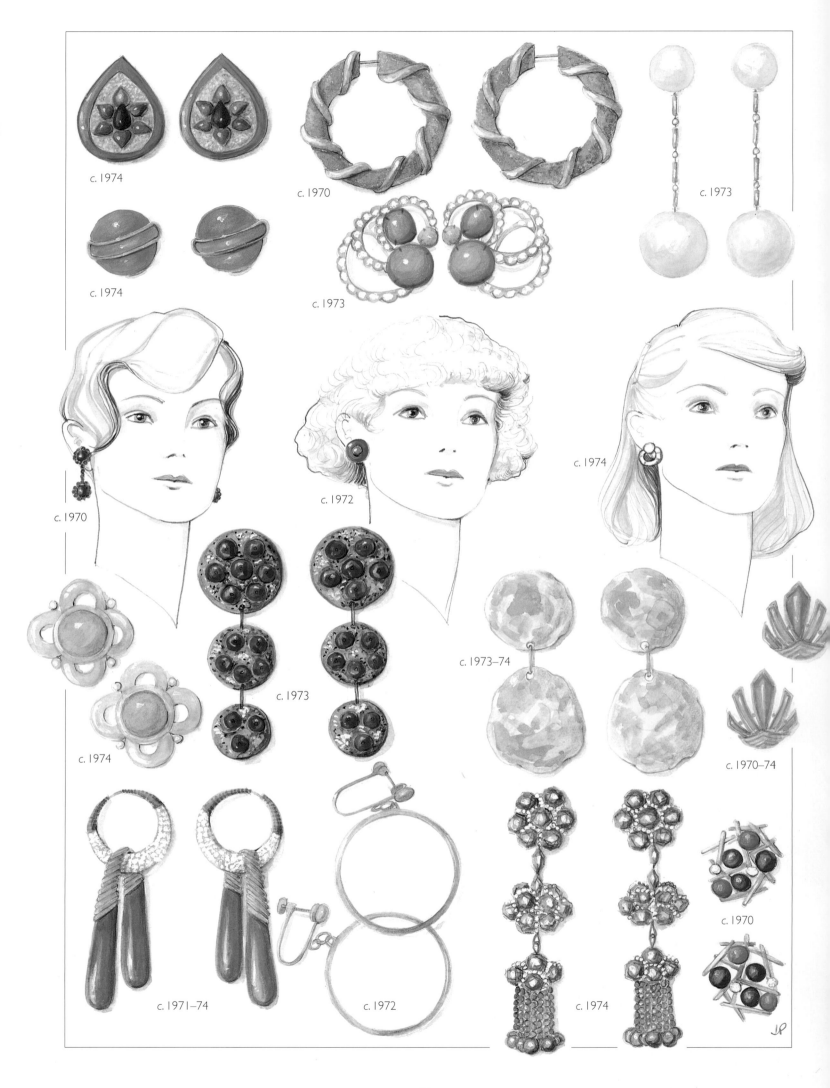

c. 1974

c. 1974

c. 1970

c. 1973

c. 1973

c. 1970

c. 1972

c. 1974

c. 1974

c. 1973

c. 1973–74

c. 1970–74

c. 1971–74

c. 1972

c. 1974

c. 1970

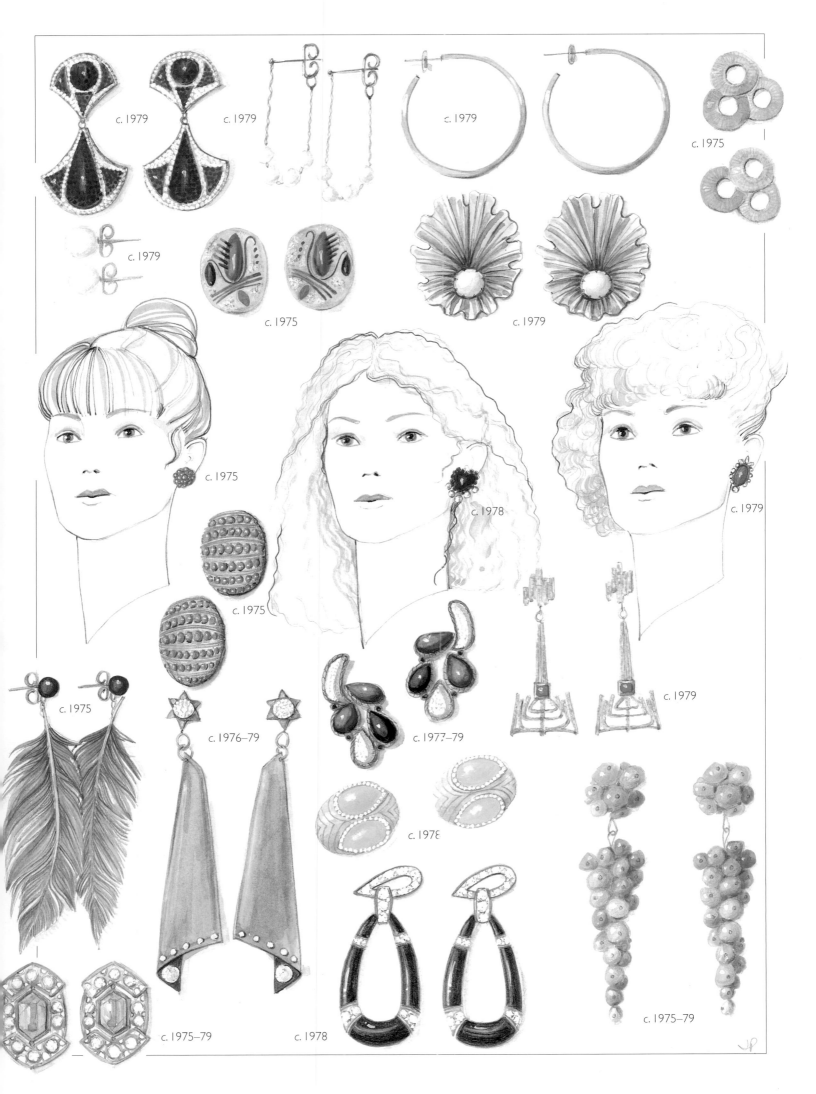

c. 1979

c. 1979

c. 1979

c. 1975

c. 1979

c. 1975

c. 1975

c. 1979

c. 1975

c. 1978

c. 1979

c. 1975

c. 1975

c. 1975

c. 1976–79

c. 1977–79

c. 1979

c. 1978

c. 1975–79

c. 1975–79

c. 1978

Rings 1970–1979

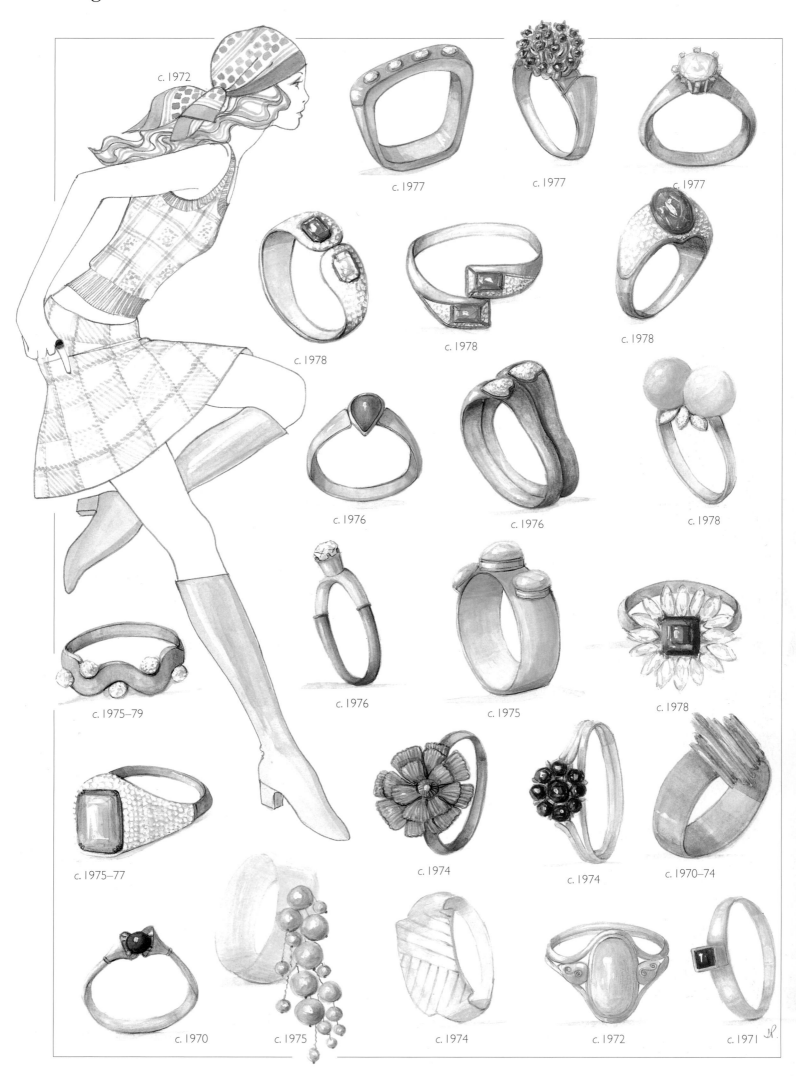

c. 1972

c. 1977

c. 1977

c. 1977

c. 1978

c. 1978

c. 1978

c. 1976

c. 1976

c. 1978

c. 1975–79

c. 1976

c. 1975

c. 1978

c. 1975–77

c. 1974

c. 1974

c. 1970–74

c. 1970

c. 1975

c. 1974

c. 1972

c. 1971

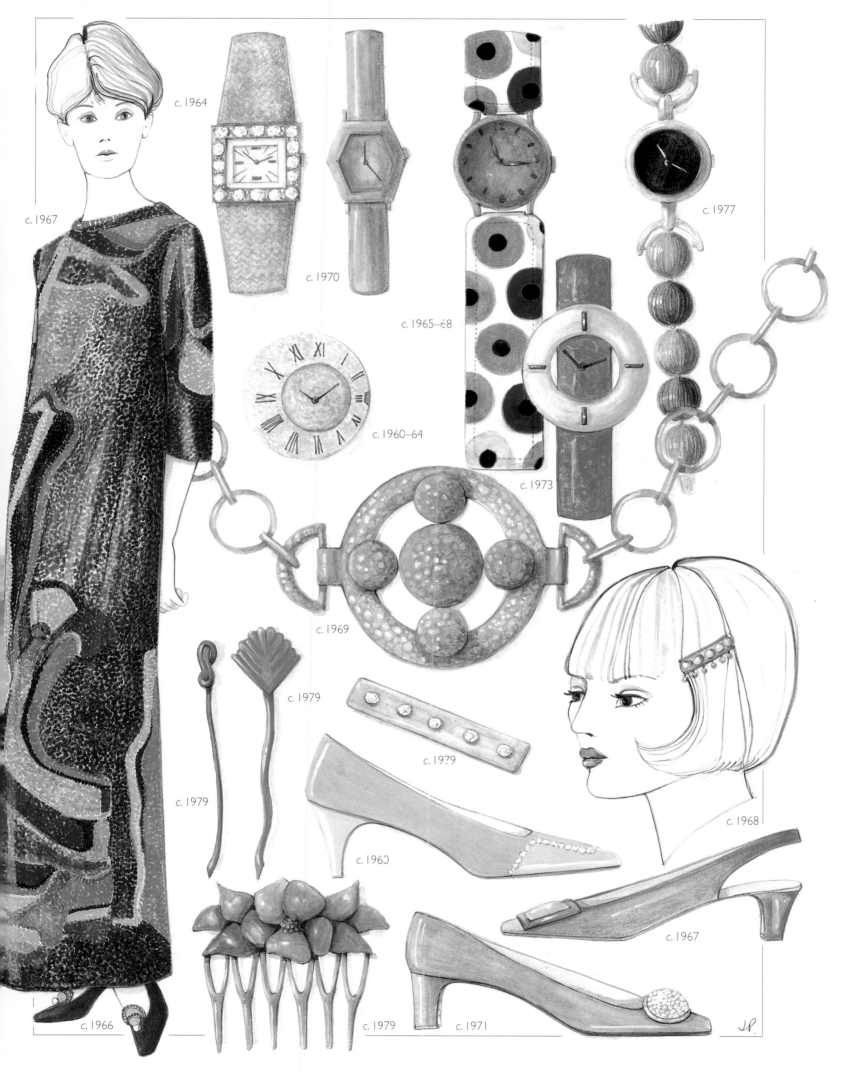

c. 1964

c. 1970

c. 1965–68

c. 1977

c. 1967

c. 1960–64

c. 1973

c. 1969

c. 1979

c. 1979

c. 1979

c. 1968

c. 1960

c. 1967

c. 1966

c. 1979

c. 1971

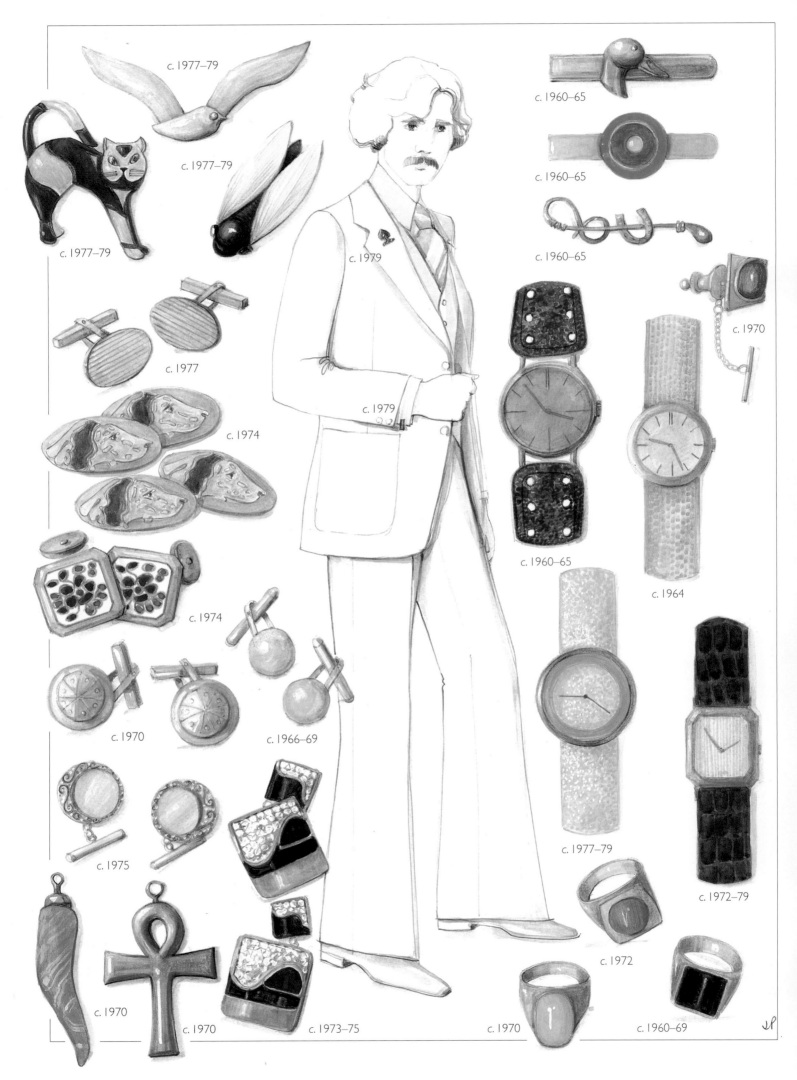

c. 1977–79

c. 1977–79

c. 1977–79

c. 1979

c. 1960–65

c. 1960–65

c. 1960–65

c. 1977

c. 1974

c. 1979

c. 1970

c. 1974

c. 1960–65

c. 1964

c. 1970

c. 1966–69

c. 1977–79

c. 1975

c. 1972–79

c. 1972

c. 1970

c. 1970

c. 1973–75

c. 1970

c. 1960–69

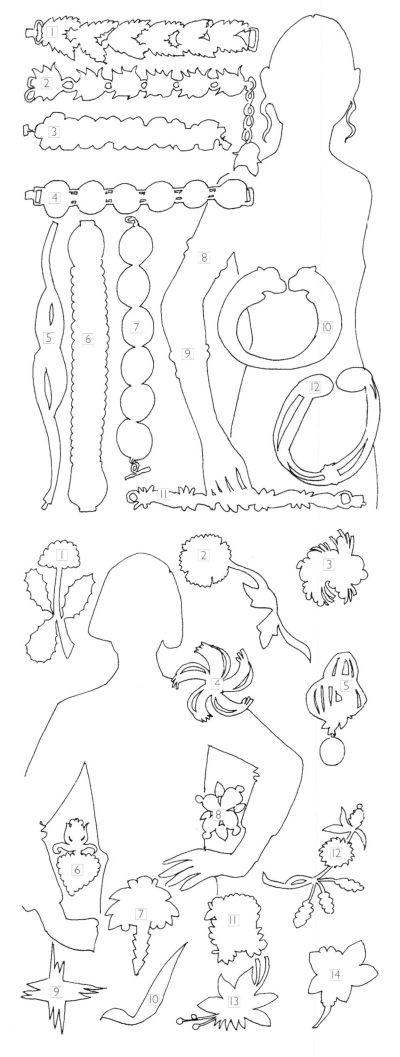

Bracelets and Bangles 1960–1969

1 c. 1960. Gilded-metal bracelet, multicoloured enamelled leaf design, set with clear paste stones on hinged joints. 2 c. 1965–68. Gilded-metal bracelet composed of open foliate-design plates, set with multicoloured moulded-glass stones, matching extended link fastening. 3 c. 1965–68. Bracelet composed of cut natural shell pieces, linked with gold-coloured chain, matching screw fastening. 4 c. 1966. Polished silver-coloured metal bracelet, decorated with papier-mâché plates, painted in Op Art design. 5 c. 1960–63. Bracelet composed of two lines of entwined and graduating brilliant-cut diamonds and emeralds, mounted in flexible setting. 6 c. 1965. Multi-strings of coloured-glass beads caught into seashell clasps decorated with paste stones. In the style of Kenneth Jay Lane. 7 c. 1969. Oxidized and polished silver linked bracelet, composed of joined split discs with 'D' design, matching silver joints and chain fastening. In the style of Patricia Meyerowitz. 8 c. 1968–69. Textured gold snake bangle. 9 c. 1968–69. Tubular gold rope bangle, hinged fastening. 10 c. 1965. Gold panther bracelet, set with diamonds, onyx spots and emerald eyes. In the style of Cartier. 11 c. 1964. Platinum bracelet, composed of floral sprays and open links set with various sized brilliant-cut diamonds. 12 c. 1960–62. Gilded-metal double-band bracelet, set with two mottled stones, decorative setting to open front, hinged back fastening.

Brooches 1960–1969

1 c. 1963. Platinum and gold floral brooch, leaves set with diamonds, clover flowerhead with cabochon sapphires. 2 c. 1960–65. Metal floral brooch, enamelled carnation flowerhead with coloured-glass stone centre, edges of petals touched with gold paint, matching stem and leaves. 3 c. 1960–65. Gold brooch, free-flowing scroll design, set with brilliant-cut diamonds. 4 c. 1965–69. Silver-coloured metal brooch, flowing, polished and textured spikes surrounding large mock pearl. 5 c. 1965–69. Platinum brooch, large pearl suspended under spray of leaf-shaped diamonds and looped ribbons set with rubies and diamonds. In the style of Chaumet. 6 c. 1960. Coloured-glass stone mounted in silver, set with rhinestones, matching asymmetric heart-shaped pendant. 7 c. 1960. Platinum brooch in palm-tree design, set with diamonds and rubies. In the style of Bulgari. 8 c. 1960–65. Gold-coloured metal brooch, comprising four pear-shaped coloured-glass stones, spaced by smaller stones, topped with clear stones. 9 c. 1960–65. Gold-coloured metal brooch, stepped cross-bar design, set with coloured cabochon stones. 10 1960–65. Gold brooch, twisted leaf-shape with pavé-set diamonds. 11 c. 1960–65. Large amethyst in platinum frame, set with random clusters of various sized diamonds. 12 c. 1965–69. Gold brooch, stylized rose spray set with brilliant-cut diamonds. 13 c. 1969. Floral brooch in textured gold, centre of flower set with single emerald within cluster of diamond stamens with emerald tips. 14 c. 1965–69. Floral brooch, centre of flower set with spray cluster of brilliant-cut diamonds, petals of pavé-set rubies, diamond-set stem.

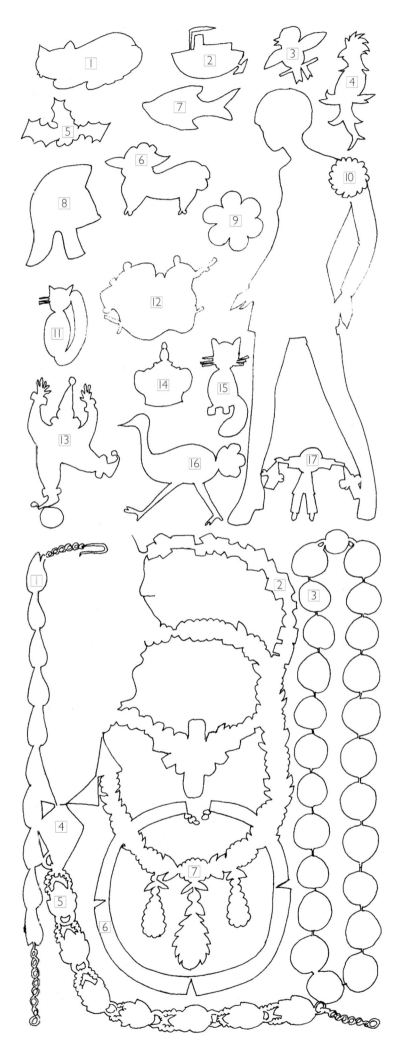

Novelty Brooches 1960–1969

1 c. 1960–64. Gold-plated silver-mesh cat brooch with enamelled eyes and detail. 2 c. 1960. Sterling-silver boat brooch set with faceted coloured-glass stones and rhinestones. 3 c. 1966. Gold-plated bird brooch set with tiny fake-turquoise beads, cabochon coloured-glass eye and matching pavé-set body. 4 c. 1968. Matt-gold parrot brooch, enamelled beak, cabochon ruby eye and cabochon emerald body. 5 c. 1960–63. Enamelled silver holly brooch, tips of two leaves set with rhinestones, synthetic cabochon ruby berries. 6 c. 1960–65. Twisted gold-coloured wire brooch, in the form of a sheep. 7 c. 1966–69. Multicoloured polished-plastic fish brooch. 8 c. 1960–65. Gold-coloured metal Roman helmet brooch, engraved detail, set with rhinestones. 9 c. 1966–69. Flower brooch composed of flat multicoloured plastic discs. 10 c. 1966. Two-colour plastic daisy brooch. 11 c. 1960. Gold-coloured metal cat brooch, fake cabochon coral head and body. 12 c. 1966–69. Gold painted metal brooch, design based on the Beatles pop group. 13 c. 1960–65. Gold-plated sterling-silver-mesh clown brooch, fake-pearl trim. 14 c. 1960–65. Gold-plated silver crown brooch, set with fake cabochon emeralds, rubies, sapphires and faceted rhinestones. In the style of Trifari. 15 c. 1969. Engraved matt-gold cat brooch, cabochon emerald body, matching single eye, diamond eyebrows. 16 c. 1965–69. Sterling-silver running ostrich brooch, set with large rhinestones and fake-ruby eye, enamelled detail to wings and tail. 17 c. 1960. Gold-plated silver Chinese flower carrier brooch, hat set with large fake pearl, enamelled costume, matching flowers in baskets suspended from fine chains.

Necklaces and Pendants 1960–1965

1 c. 1960–62. Silver-coloured metal choker necklace, foliate design set with shaped two-tone plastic stones, chain back, hook fastening. 2 c. 1960. Short necklace, set with multicoloured synthetic stones, central pendant section set with larger matching stones, scroll and openwork spacers set with synthetic diamonds, concealed back fastening. 3 c. 1960–62. Long plastic-bead necklace, each bead sliced into sections forming stripes in three colours, brass wire links, matching clip fastening and fixings. 4 c. 1965. Fine gold wire necklace, composed of triangular plates, openwork-lace design, linked by fine gold rings, matching pendant of two facing plates overlaid with beaten gold-leaf leaves, chain back. 5 c. 1960–64. Gold-coloured choker necklace, foliate design set with pale-coloured shaped plastic stones, linked by large rings and half-wreaths, chain back. 6 c. 1965. Choker necklace, composed of four graduated shaped copper plaques, multicoloured abstract enamelled decoration, linked by copper rings on top edge, matching chain and clasp fastening. 7 c. 1962. Platinum necklace, floral plaques set with large cushion-cut emeralds surrounded by brilliant-cut diamonds, matching articulated foliate spacers and three pendant drops to front of necklace, concealed back fastening. In the style of Van Cleef & Arpels.

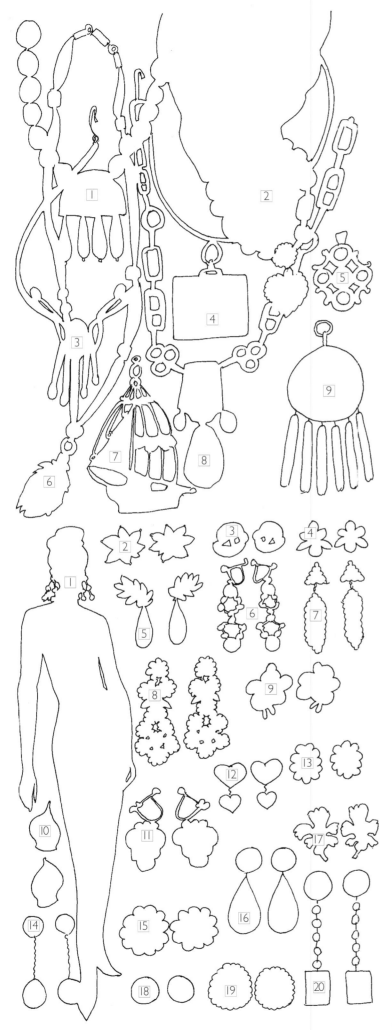

Necklaces and Pendants 1965–1969

1 c. 1958. Marbled stone bead necklace, matching elongated pear-shaped drops on lower edge of semicircular gold-coloured metal pendant decorated with stone beads. 2 c. 1968. Long necklace composed of carved ruby, emerald and sapphire beads, diamond trim, matching narrow spacers, central clasp fastening and heart-shaped pendant. In the style of Van Cleef & Arpels. 3 c. 1965. Flexible gold rope necklace, large faceted coloured stone in centre, matching similar smaller stones on tips of rope pendants. 4 c. 1965–69. Rigid silver-coloured wire choker with large square pendant plaque in matching material, engraved sunburst design around central domed plastic stone. 5 c. 1969. Silver pendant composed of mottled semi-precious stone surrounded by openwork discs and half discs. 6 c. 1965–69. Multicoloured silk cord necklace, random knots with coloured-glass bead covers, multicoloured feather pendant, polished-brass fixing, matching screw fastening. 7 c. 1965. Gold-coloured metal galleon pendant, raised and engraved decoration and detail, fine metal chain trim. 8 c. 1969. Yellow-gold-coloured metal necklace, composed of openwork cast plates with flexible links, multi-piece pendant, pierced design random set with semi-precious turquoise-coloured stones, hook fastening. 9 c. 1965–69. Large metal disc pendant, multicoloured enamel, design of stylized waterlilies, enamelled pendant fringe.

Earrings 1960–1969

1 c. 1967. Outsized gold-coloured plastic clip-on pendant earrings, composed of balls studded with tiny rhinestones, matching tiny coloured ball spacers with chain links. 2 c. 1960–64. Openwork clip-on earrings, gold-coloured metal framework set with faceted clear paste stones. 3 c. 1960–65. Free-flowing scroll-design gold clip-on earrings, set with lines of brilliant-cut diamonds. 4 c. 1960. Pearl-look-plastic foliate-design clip-on earrings. 5 c. 1968. Platinum foliate-design earrings, set with diamonds and pale-pink coral, matching teardrop pendants. In the style of Asprey & Co. 6 c. 1962–65. Pendant earrings set with coloured-glass stones, set in gold-coloured metal, screw fastenings. 7 c. 1966. Pendant earrings set with polished stones, angular design. In the style of Swarovski. 8 c. 1965–69. Outsized pendant earrings, floral-wreath design, rubies surrounded by diamonds. In the style of Van Cleef & Arpels. 9 c. 1960–65. Pierced gold-coloured metal frame set with various sized black and white beads. 10 c. 1965–68. Shell clip-on earrings, mounted in gold wire, set with coral. 11 c. 1960. Gold-coloured metal pendant earrings, set with marbled-glass stones, screw fastenings. 12 c. 1969. Plastic heart-shaped clip-on earrings, set with faceted glass stone, heart-shaped gold plastic pendant. 13 c. 1960–65. Cabochon sapphire clip-on earrings, brilliant-cut diamond surround. 14 c. 1965. Gold-coloured plastic clip-on earrings, ball and chain pendants. 15 c. 1960–65. Plastic bead clip-on earrings. 16 c. 1962–64. Plastic pendant earrings, decorated with coloured sequins. In the style of Kenneth Jay Lane. 17 c. 1960–65. Gold clip-on earrings, foliate design set with coloured stones. 18 c. 1964–68. Painted papier-mâché earrings. 19 c. 1965. Openwork clip-on earrings set with diamonds and emeralds. 20 c. 1965–69. Two-colour plastic clip-on pendant earrings.

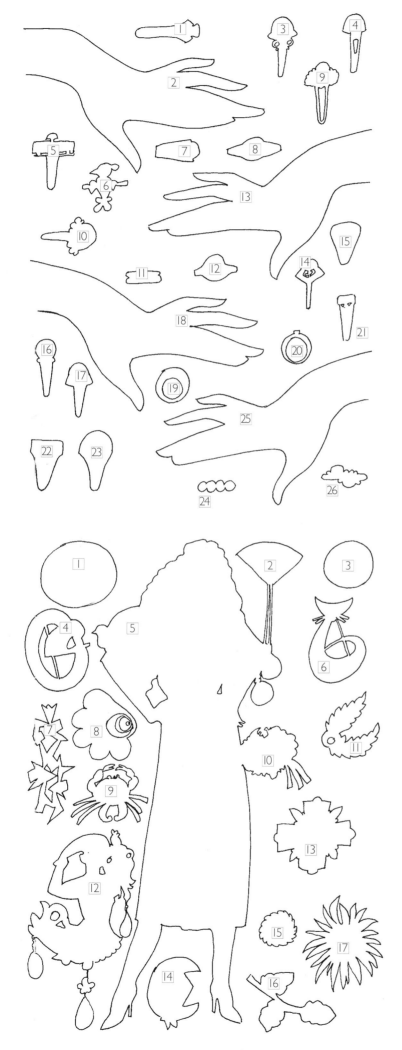

Rings 1960–1969

1 *c.* 1960. Platinum ring, set with sapphires, pavé-set diamond shoulders. 2 *c.* 1965. Marquise-shaped diamond ring. 3 *c.* 1960–65. Polished semi-precious stone in decorative gilded-metal mount, matching open shoulders. 4 *c.* 1960–65. Gold-coloured metal ring, engraved self-metal 'stone', open shoulders. 5 *c.* 1965. Silver ring, coloured stone set with matching decorative scroll. 6 *c.* 1965–69. Stylized bird ring, multicoloured semi-precious stones set in silver. 7 *c.* 1960–65. Silver ring with latticework shoulders, central glass stone, flower design under surface. 8 *c.* 1960–65. Gilded-metal r ng, latticework shoulders and back, coloured-glass stone with white pattern under surface. 9 *c.* 1960–65. Silver ring, chrysanthemum design, pearl centre, open shoulders. 10 *c.* 1969. Gold-coloured metal ring, large coloured stone with surround of graded coloured beads. 11 *c.* 1969. Two-tier mock-ivory ring set with clear faceted stones. 12 *c.* 1965–69. Silver ring, flat central disc set with coloured stone. 13 *c.* 1969. Ruby and diamond ring, flat face and wide shoulders. 14 *c.* 1968. Gold ring, cabochon ruby set above winged shoulders and gold balls. 15 *c.* 1969. Flared band, engraved and set with brilliant-cut diamonds. 16 *c.* 1965–69. Engraved gold ring set with fake pearl. 17 *c.* 1965–69. Synthetic cabochon emerald, fancy mount, matching shoulders. 18 *c.* 1969. Wide band set with four rows of black and white fake pearls. 19 *c.* 1966–69. Mock-ivory ring, set with faceted stones, gilt back. 20 *c.* 1966–69. Black plastic ring, central rhinestone, gilt insets. 21 *c.* 1969. Gold ring, cushion-cut stone, matching smaller stones in open shoulders. 22 *c.* 1968. One-piece moulded-plastic ring, grad.ated colour. 23 *c.* 1967–69. One-piece moulded-plastic ring, Japanese-style painted face under clear dome. 24 *c.* 1965–69. Pearls and turquoise stones set in gold wire framework. 25 *c.* 1969. Synthetic cabochon ruby, surround of black and white pearls. 26 *c.* 1969. Gold band decorated with fake pearls.

Brooches 1970–1979

1 *c.* 1974–78. Round plastic brooch comprising a framed portrait of a 1970s-style girl wearing a cloche hat over long, curled hair. 2 *c.* 1975. Triangular copper brooch, multicoloured enamel decoration, matching flat discs topped with coloured-glass beads suspended from fine wires. 3 *c.* 1975. Silver disc brooch, raised mythical-animal design against polished background. 4 *c.* 1975–79. Engraved and polished silver brooch, open abstract design. 5 *c.* 1975–79. Gold-coloured metal stylized bird brooch set with multicoloured glass stones and mock-mother-of-pearl insets. 6 *c.* 1970. Polished-steel stylized cat brooch. 7 *c.* 1975–79. Engraved silver brooch comprising interlocking arrow-shaped plaques set with square synthetic emeralds. 8 *c.* 1975. Foliate-design silver slip brooch, textured leaves with polished edges and stems. 9 *c.* 1970–75. Gold crab brooch, pierced diamond-set body with central cabochon ruby, matching legs and claws, cabochon sapphire eyes. 10 *c.* 1970–75. Gold floral brooch, central cluster of emeralds set within a pierced spray of diamond set petals, stems set with baguette diamonds. 11 *c.* 1975. Fern-leaf brooch, two-colour gold fronds set with diamonds. 12 *c.* 1974. Renaissance-style brooch, multicoloured enamel decoration, fake ruby, sapphire and emerald trim, man-fish with fake-pearl body, matching baroque pearl drops. In the style of Hattie Carnegie. 13 *c.* 1970–75. Gold wire cross brooch, set with various sized cabochon rubies and turquoise stones. 14 *c.* 1975. Painted plastic man-in-the-moon Pierrot brooch. In the style of Butler & Wilson. 15 *c.* 1979. Mock-turquoise stone set in decorative gold-coloured metal mount. 16 *c.* 1975. Foliate-design copper brooch, enamelled branch and stylized leaves. In the style of Matisse. 17 *c.* 1979. Faceted coloured-glass stone in gold-coloured metal prong setting, irregular sunburst surround, small rays set with tiny matching stones.

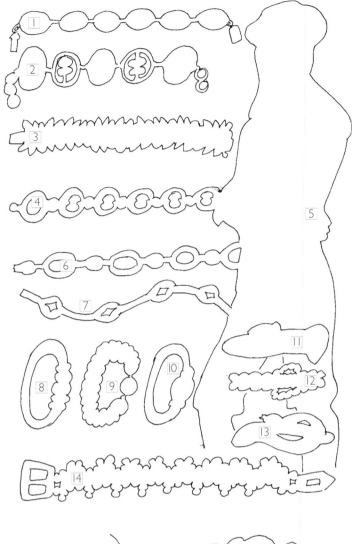

Bracelets and Bangles 1970–1979

1 *c.* 1970. Silver bracelet, composed of oval plaques decorated with multicoloured enamels, silver chain links. 2 *c.* 1970–75. Silver bracelet, composed of three oval plaques set with mock-turquoise stones, open disc spacers, two small mock-turquoise stones set with fake rubies suspended from silver chain within each centre, silver links and fastening. 3 *c.* 1975. Rectangular emerald stones surrounded by diamonds form plaques linked by flexible platinum rods, matching fastening. 4 *c.* 1970–75. Bracelet composed of open circular coral plaques, gold and cabochon ruby spacing links. 5 *c.* 1975. Multicoloured shiny plastic bangles. 6 *c.* 1970–75. Textured-gold bracelet, composed of oval open discs, linking bars set with oval cabochon onyx. 7 *c.* 1975–79. Plaited yellow-gold wire bracelet, open-knot design. In the style of Boucheron. 8 *c.* 1975–79. Gold-coloured metal bangle set with faceted clear glass stones, matching bars between and either side the twisted plastic rods in the front section concealing opening. 9 *c.* 1978. Multicoloured twisted ropes of fake pearls, gilt plastic coral and faceted clear glass stops either side carved plastic ball concealing fastening. 10 *c.* 1975–79. Plastic bangle, front detail set with clear and coloured faceted plastic stones, gilt trim, matching back fastening. 11 *c.* 1970–74. Gold bangle, leopard-head design, fine enamel decoration set with diamonds. In the style of Jean Eté. 12 *c.* 1977. Twisted-gold bangle, interlocked loop at front set with brilliant-cut diamonds. In the style of Boucheron. 13 *c.* 1970–74. Gold snake bangle, fine enamel set with small parels of diamonds. In the style of Jean Eté. 14 *c.* 1970–75. Plastic-bead bracelet, glued and threaded bead plaques spaced by gilt rods, matching buckle fastening.

Necklaces and Pendants 1970–1974

1 *c.* 1971. Large two-tone shiny plastic beads form back of long necklace, silk tassel pendant under single matching bead and row of smaller beads, matching pendant earrings. 2 *c.* 1970. Two-tier gold pendant set with pink and green cabochon synthetic stones suspended from double-plaited gold chain spaced with matching coloured beads. In the style of Van Cleef & Arpels. 3 *c.* 1972. Ceramic collar and matching pendant, composed of rectangular plaques glazed in two colours, flower pattern with gold-coloured metal centres, matching outsized chain links, concealed front fastening above pendant. 4 *c.* 1972. Silver choker composed of engraved open plaques forming knots, with continuous twisted rope effect, concealed fastening. 5 *c.* 1974. Oblong pendant, mottled pink stone held in wavy asymmetric silver frame. 6 *c.* 1974. Circular silver pendant, design of swimming fish around central pond of mother-of-pearl. 7 *c.* 1973. Silver pendant, asymmetric abstract design, large flat silver plate balanced by faceted coloured-glass stone. 8 *c.* 1973. Large gold pendant, floral design set with outsized cabochon sapphires and surrounded by diamonds, leaf-shaped sprays set with various sized and shaped cabochon emeralds, gold chain-link back spaced with similar motifs set with matching gems. In the style of Boucheron. 9 *c.* 1973. Mottled glaze ceramic head, brushed with gold and decorated with fake-pearl bead drops, suspended from plaited silk cord threaded with matching flat ceramic beads, loop and flat bead fastening.

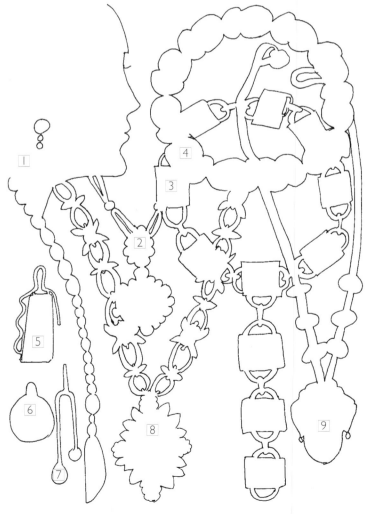

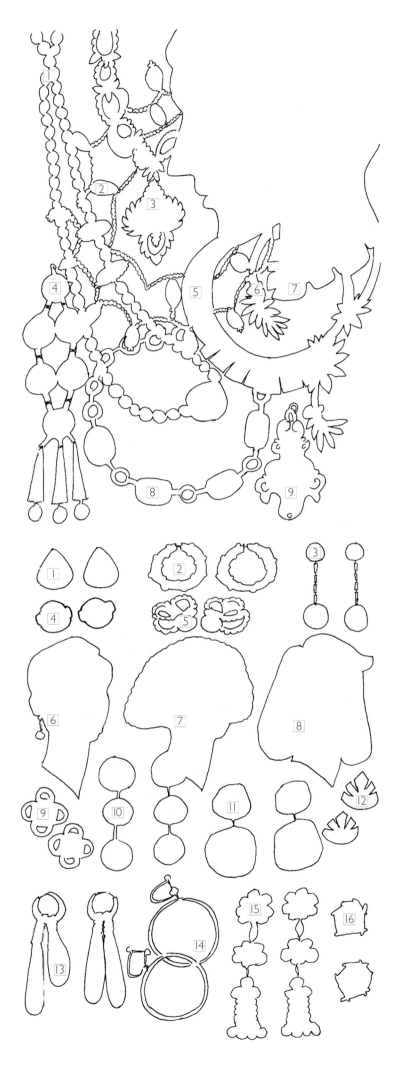

Necklaces and Pendants 1975–1979

1 c. 1975. Ridged plastic-bead necklace, long strand with outsized plastic pearl threaded in centre. 2 c. 1978. Gold necklace, composed of two scalloped bars set with diamonds linked and edged with polished coral set top and bottom with large diamonds. In the style of Boucheron. 3 c. 1977. Gold pendant, linked-leaf design set with diamonds, shape emphasized with sapphires, necklace of matching design set with similar stones. 4 c. 1975. Silver-coloured metal pendant, composed of linked discs, engraved floral design, matching fringe trim with polished ball drops. 5 c. 1977. Multicoloured-gem-set gold collar, composed of square collets set with citrine, garnet, tourmaline, amethyst, iolite, aquamarine and peridot. In the style of Andrew Grima. 6 c. 1978. Flexible plaited-gold wire necklace, open asymmetric design, decorated with sprays of flowers, petals set with diamonds, onyx centres and buds. 7 c. 1979. Short gold necklace, two sizes of half-moon-shaped plaques, multicoloured enamel decoration set with diamonds, diamond and fine gold chain spacers. 8 c. 1979. Gold choker, oval plaques set with large octagonal emeralds surrounded by diamonds, matching diamond-set open links and spacers. In the style of Bulgari. 9 c. 1975. Textured gold-coloured metal pendant, flexible pierced scroll design, highlighted with polished gold-coloured balls, fine hinges between upper and lower motifs.

Earrings 1970–1974

1 c. 1974. Leaf-shaped clip-on earrings, enamelled border, matching raised pattern against textured-gold background. 2 c. 1970. Large gold hoop earrings, textured background with coiled polished ribbon detail. 3 c. 1973. Large fake-pearl balls suspended from line of glass beads under pearl studs. 4 c. 1974. Round plastic clip-on earrings, gilt trim. 5 c. 1973. Gold clip-on earrings, open-loop design, scalloped edges set with diamonds, decorated with cluster of sapphires, emeralds and peridots. 6 c. 1970. Fake cabochon ruby earrings, surrounded by small shiny black stones, matching pendants. 7 c. 1972. Large two-colour plastic disc clip-on earrings. 8 c. 1974. Gold earrings, half-circular hoops set with diamonds, single diamond studs. 9 c. 1974. Silver clip-on earrings, central cabochon stone with surround of open loops and beads. 10 c. 1973. Textured-black-plastic clip-on earrings, flat discs touched with gold paint and trimmed with sequins, matching smaller disc pendants. 11 c. 1973–74. Pressed gold-coloured metal clip-on earrings, matching large pendants. 12 c. 1970–74. Gold-coloured metal clip-on earrings, set with coral-coloured plastic stones. 13 c. 1971–74. Asymmetric hoop earrings, front set with diamonds, back covered with twisted gold wire, matching covers of polished-coral pendants. 14 c. 1972. Outsized polished-gold hoops, suspended from small studs with screw fastenings. 15 c. 1974. Floral earrings, faceted plastic beads spaced by strings of tiny sparkling beads, matching pendants with fringed bead tassel. 16 c. 1970. Gold clip-on earrings, stick design set with cabochon emeralds, rubies, sapphires and brilliant-cut diamonds.

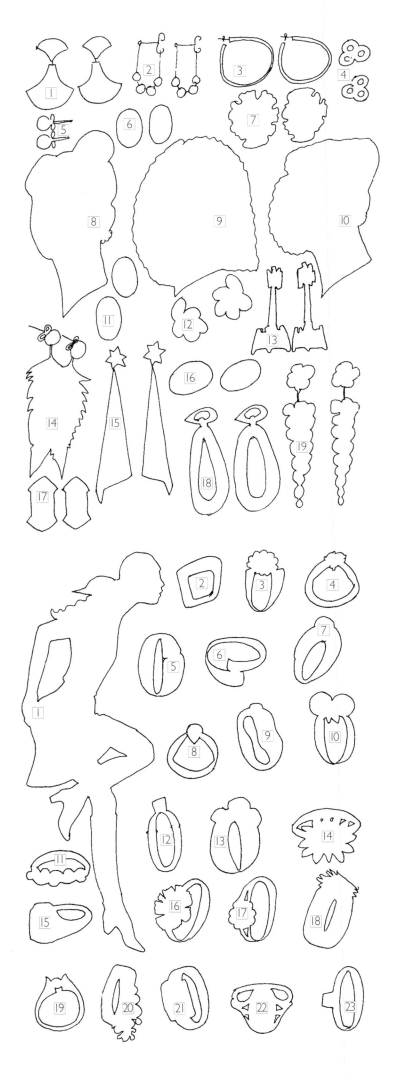

Earrings 1975–1979

1 c. 1979. Pendant earrings, all-over mosaic pattern of clear and coloured plastic stones. 2 c. 1979. Row of four small pearls linked by and suspended from fine gold chain. 3 c. 1979. Outsized split gold hoop earrings. 4 c. 1975. Three-colour textured-gold earrings, composed of overlaid open hoops. 5 c. 1979. Gold pierced pearl studs. 6 c. 1975. Painted ceramic clip-on earrings, abstract design. 7 c. 1979. Pressed fine gold-coloured metal outsized clip-on earrings, leaf design, prong-set single fake pearl in centre. 8 c. 1975. Plastic bead cluster clip-on earrings. 9 c. 1978. Outsized clip-on earrings, heart-shaped glass ruby surrounded by gold-coloured beads, base fringed with clear glass pendants. 10 c. 1979. Outsized clip-on earrings, oval cabochon fake sapphire set in gold frame, surrounded by fake diamonds. 11 c. 1975. Gold clip-on earrings, oval shape ridged and set with turquoise stones. 12 c. 1977–79. Clip-on earrings, twisted gold wire leaf-shaped frames set with cabochon coral, onyx and brilliant-cut diamonds. 13 c. 1979. Textured gold-coloured metal pendant earrings, abstract design set with single fake emerald. 14 c. 1975. Feather suspended from pierced plastic stud. 15 c. 1976–79. Plastic handkerchief pendants set with rhinestones, suspended from star-shaped studs set with similar stones. 16 c. 1978. Engraved gold oval clip-on earrings set with pale-coloured coral surrounded by diamonds. 17 c. 1975–79. Gold earrings, pierced design set with single sapphire with diamond surround. 18 c. 1978. Open leaf-shaped mock-onyx pendants banded with gold-coloured plastic set with sparkling stones, matching stud and links. 19 c. 1975–79. Cluster of misshapen transparent plastic beads form studs above elongated tapered pendants.

Rings 1970–1979

1 c. 1972. Silver ring with three-colour striped stone. 2 c. 1977. Rounded-square gold ring set with row of diamonds. 3 c. 1977. Platinum ring set with cluster of rubies on stalks. 4 c. 1977. Gold ring, single sapphire in outsized claw setting. 5 c. 1978. Gold ring, single rectangular diamond and ruby set each side centre division, diamond surround, wide shoulders. 6 c. 1978. Gold ring, crossover front, set with raised rectangular emeralds and diamond detail. 7 c. 1978. Gold ring, diamond-set flared shoulders, central cabochon sapphire. 8 c. 1976. Silver ring, leaf-shaped cabochon stone. 9 c. 1976. Two-gold ring, wavy sides, heart-shaped diamond detail. 10 c. 1978. Gold ring, black and white pearls above diamond-set leaves. 11 c. 1975–79. Gold ring, brilliant-cut diamonds set within scallops on front edge. 12 c. 1976. Two-gold ring, brilliant-cut diamond set into deep collar. 13 c. 1975. Wide silver band, three polished coloured-glass stones set into shallow collars. 14 c. 1978. Gold ring, floral design composed of large cushion-shaped ruby surrounded by diamond petals. 15 c. 1975–77. Gold-coloured metal ring, flared shoulders set with seed pearls, claw-set fake-amber stone. 16 c. 1974. Gold ring, floral design, engraved petals, bead centre set with small diamond. 17 c. 1974. Gold wire ring, floral design of garnets. 18 c. 1970–74. Gold band decorated with asymmetric textured plaque. 19 c. 1970. Gold-coloured metal ring, split front, claw-set coloured-glass stone. 20 c. 1975. Wide gold-coloured metal band, front decorated with tassel of various sized beads in same metal. 21 c. 1974. Silver ring, engraved rectangular plaque made in one piece with narrow back. 22 c. 1972. Large marbled coloured-glass stone set within pierced silver wire frame. 23 c. 1971. Silver ring, square stone glued into deep collar on front.

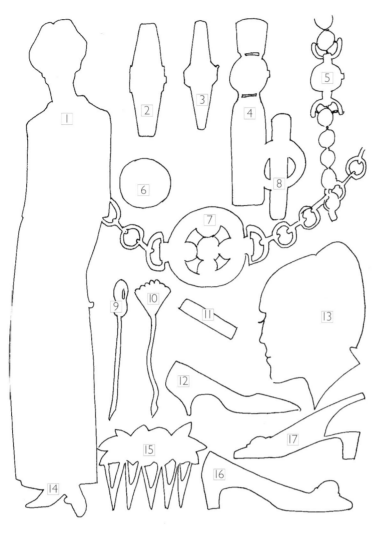

Miscellaneous Jewelry and Jewelled Pieces 1960–1979

1 c. 1967. Silk semi-fitted ankle-length evening dress, encrusted with tiny multicoloured glass beads in an abstract design. In the style of Pierre Cardin. 2 c. 1964. Wristwatch, small face, gold frame set with brilliant-cut diamonds, basket-weave bracelet strap. 3 c. 1970. Gold wristwatch, hexagonal face, no numerals, deep polished frame, matching bangle-style strap. 4 c. 1965–68. Gold-coloured metal wristwatch, matching numerals on coloured round face, wide plastic strap printed with multicoloured spots. 5 c. 1977. Wristwatch with round onyx face, no numerals, plain polished frame, matching shoulders to carved coral and onyx bead strap. 6 c. 1960–64. Two-colour gold brooch or pendant watch, textured frame set with graded roman numerals surrounding asymmetrically set inner face containing hands. 7 c. 1969. Hip belt, hammered-pewter central motif, matching half-circle side links, polished link-and-bar back. 8 c. 1973. Textured-plastic bangle wristwatch, open disc of polished metal with four coloured numeral points above hands set onto bangle. 9 c. 1979. Coloured-plastic hairpin, elongated knot-design head. 10 c. 1979. Coloured-plastic hairpin, scalloped fan-shaped design head. 11 c. 1979. Polished-gold hairslide/barrette set with five brilliant-cut diamonds. 12 c. 1960. Two-tone leather shoes, shaped toecaps edged with rhinestones. 13 c. 1968. Gold-coloured metal hairslide/barrette, bar set with coral-coloured stones, lower edge with fringe of gold-coloured beads. 14 c. 1966. Silk evening shoes decorated with two tiny wired silk fans edged with gold beads, central fake pearl. 15 c. 1979. Coloured-plastic haircomb, design of flowers and stems. 16 c. 1971. Black silk evening shoes, fronts trimmed with domed round buckles set with sparkling stones within silver frame. 17 c. 1967. Sling-back shoes, fronts trimmed with gold-coloured metal buckles set with large coloured-plastic stone.

Men's Jewelry 1960–1979

1 c. 1977–79. Cat tie or lapel pin, gold-coloured metal decorated with multicoloured enamels. 2 c. 1977–79. Bird tie or lapel pin, polished-gold body, set with single diamond eye. 3 c. 1977–79. Moth tie or lapel pin, two-tone amber-coloured plastic. 4 c. 1979. Club-design tie or lapel pin, gold-coloured metal set with coloured-glass stones. 5 c. 1960–65. Polished-copper tie-clip, central duck's head. 6 c. 1960–65. Silver tie-clip, pierced disc decorated with multicoloured enamels. 7 c. 1977. Gold oval cufflinks, engraved striped design, rigid swivel links. 8 c. 1960–65. Gold tiepin, horseshoe and whip design. 9 c. 1970. Silver tie-stud set with coloured stone, safety chain and link. 10 c. 1974. Oval cufflinks, multicoloured enamelled dog's-head design, chain links. 11 c. 1979. Bulldog-clip-design gold cufflinks. 12 c. 1960–65. Wristwatch, gold case and numerals, textured-leather strap, punched-hole decoration. 13 c. 1964. Wristwatch, gold case, face and numerals, matching expanding strap. 14 c. 1974. Gold cufflinks, floral design in multicoloured enamels, chain links. 15 c. 1970. Silver cufflinks, raised centres, rigid swivel links. 16 c. 1966–69. Stainless-steel cufflinks, solid balls with rigid swivel links. 17 c. 1977–79. Wristwatch, round case, enamelled frame, textured-silver face, no numerals, matching bracelet strap. 18 c. 1972–79. Wristwatch, octagonal gold frame, striped face, no numerals, snakeskin strap. 19 c. 1975. Gold cufflinks, asymmetric polished centres, engraved borders. 20 c. 1973–75. Gold cufflinks, large plaques decorated with enamels and set with diamonds. 21 c. 1970. Polished-marbled-stone pendant tusk, suspended from gold fitting. 22 c. 1970. Gold pendant, ancient ankh design. 23 c. 1970. Gold ring, large opal set between wide flared shoulders. 24 c. 1972. Gold ring, flat round stone set flush with raised plaque between wide flared shoulders. 25 c. 1960–69. Gold ring, flat square onyx set flush between wide flared shoulders.

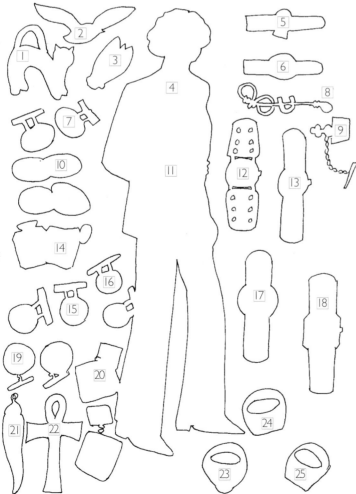

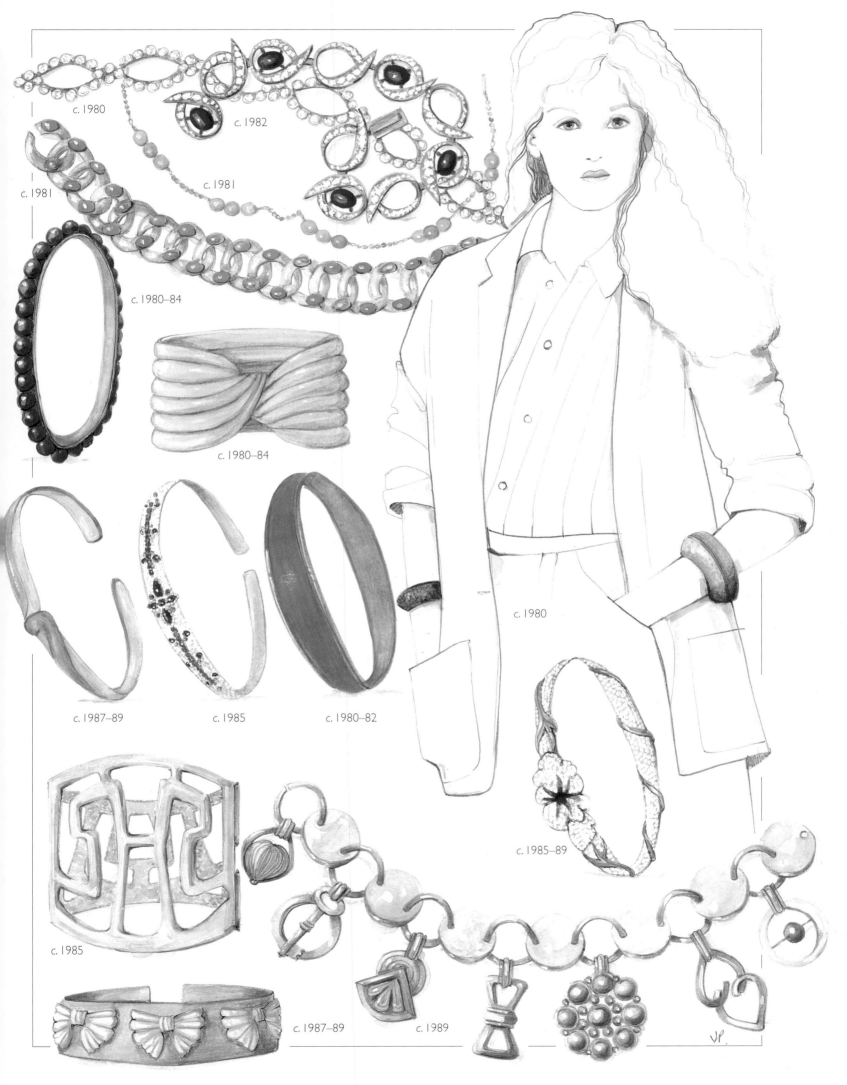

c. 1980

c. 1982

c. 1981

c. 1981

c. 1980–84

c. 1980

c. 1980–84

c. 1987–89

c. 1985

c. 1980–82

c. 1985

c. 1985–89

c. 1987–89

c. 1989

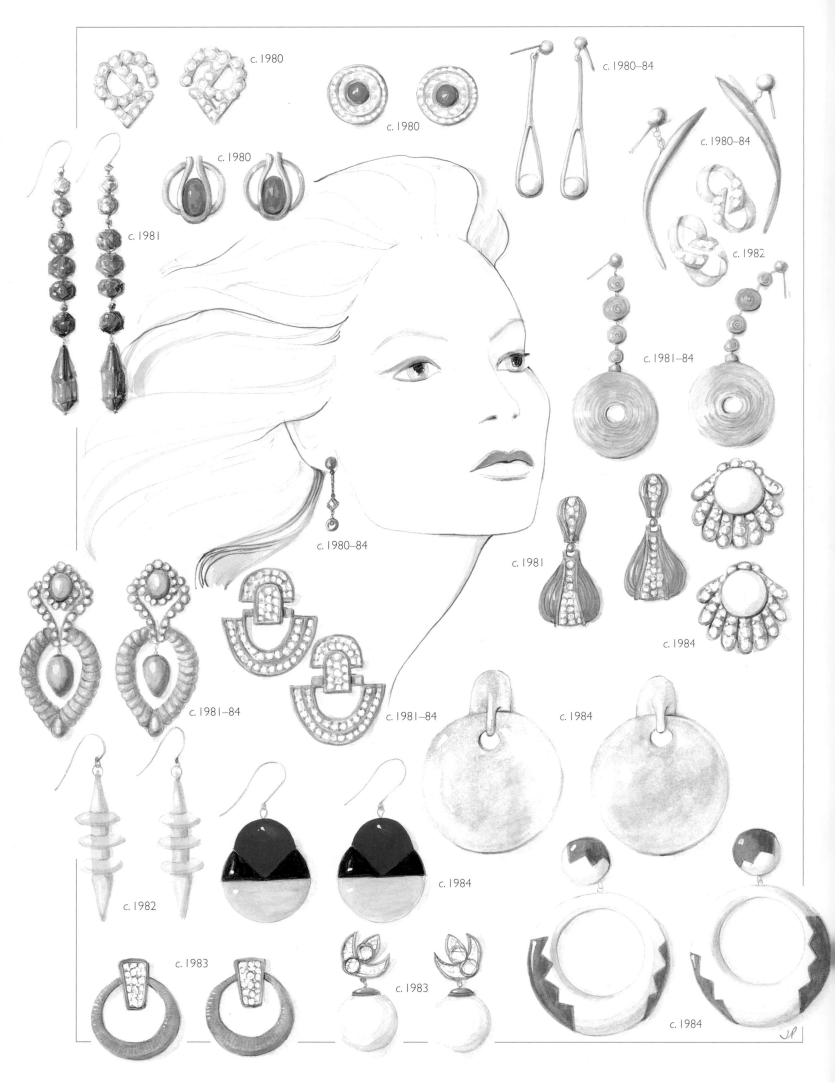

c. 1980

c. 1980

c. 1980–84

c. 1980–84

c. 1980

c. 1981

c. 1982

c. 1981–84

c. 1980–84

c. 1981

c. 1981–84

c. 1981–84

c. 1984

c. 1984

c. 1982

c. 1984

c. 1983

c. 1983

c. 1984

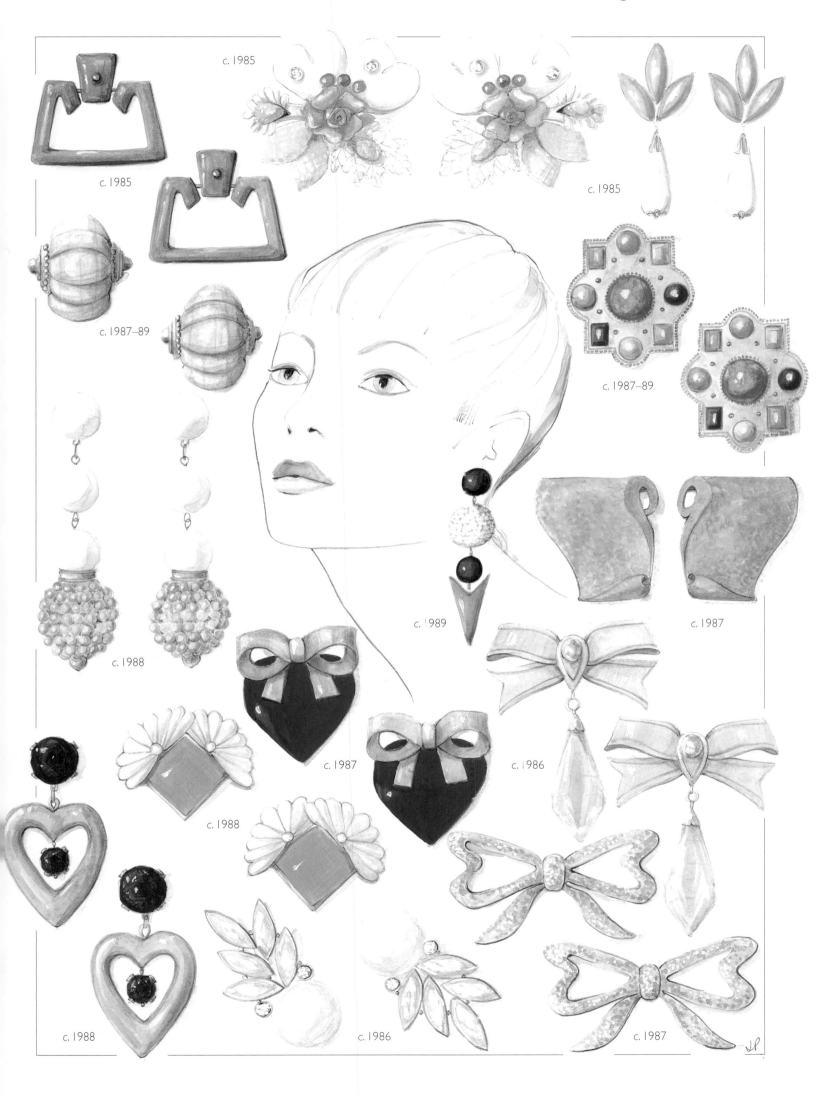

c. 1985

c. 1985

c. 1985

c. 1985

c. 1987–89

c. 1987–89

c. 1987

c. 1989

c. 1988

c. 1988

c. 1987

c. 1986

c. 1988

c. 1988

c. 1986

c. 1987

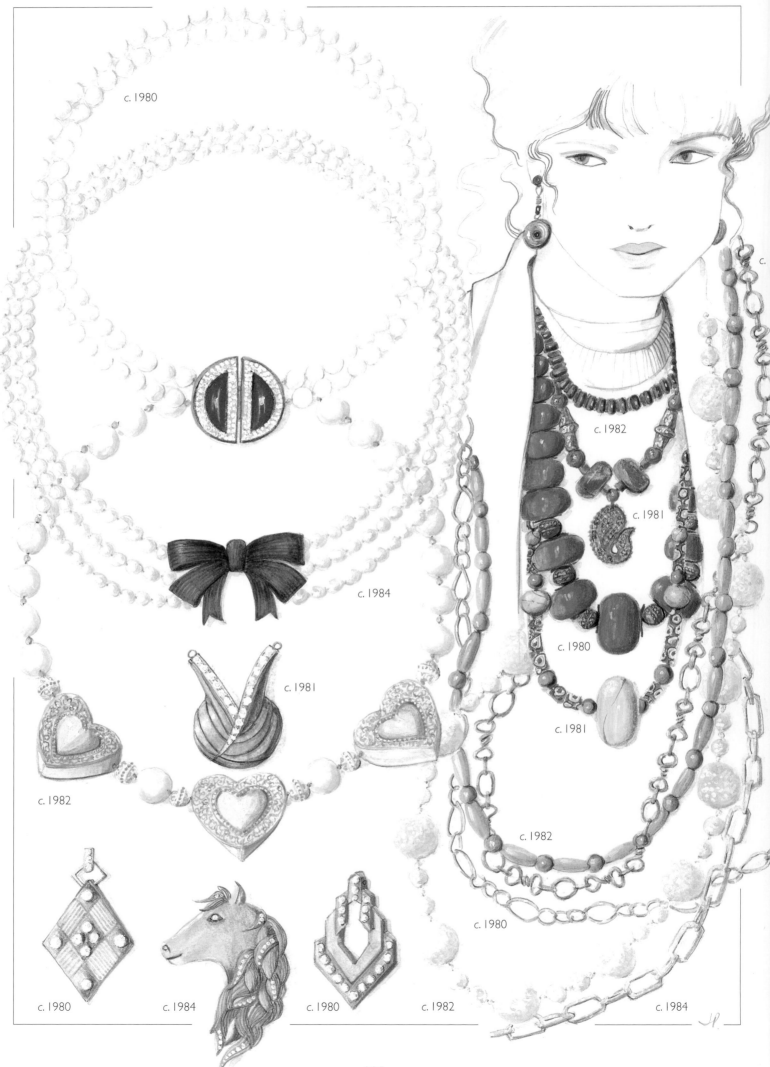

c. 1980

c. 1984

c. 1981

c. 1982

c. 1982

c. 1980

c. 1984

c. 1980

c. 1982

c. 1982

c. 1981

c. 1980

c. 1981

c. 1982

c. 1980

c.

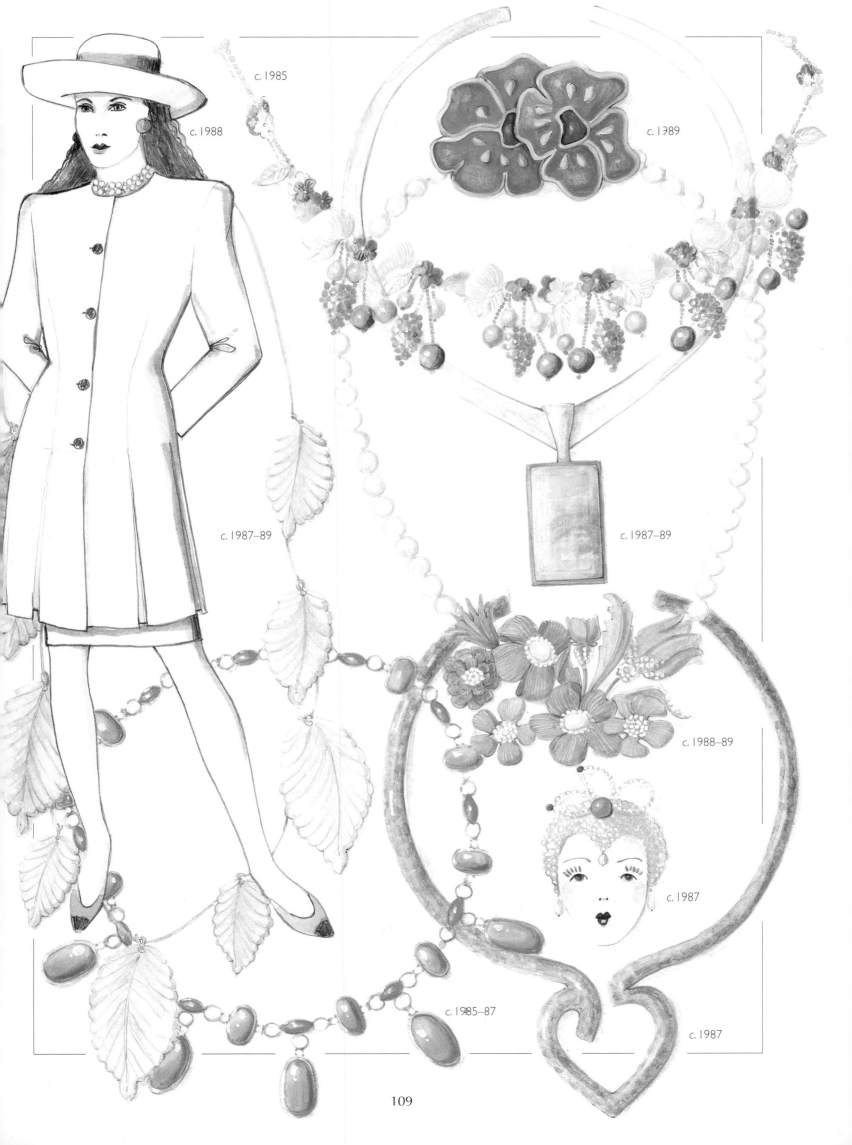

c.1985

c.1988

c.1989

c.1987–89

c.1987–89

c.1988–89

c.1987

c.1985–87

c.1987

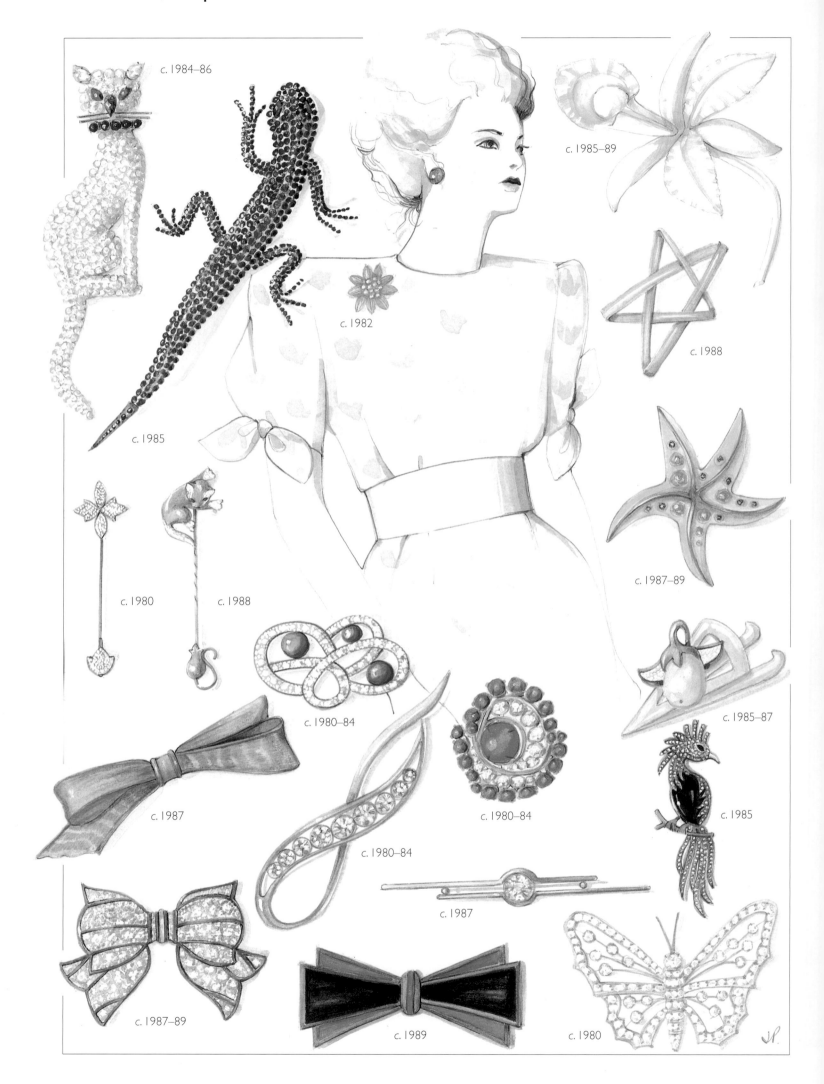

c. 1984–86

c. 1985–89

c. 1982

c. 1985

c. 1988

c. 1980

c. 1988

c. 1987–89

c. 1980–84

c. 1985–87

c. 1987

c. 1980–84

c. 1985

c. 1980–84

c. 1987

c. 1987–89

c. 1989

c. 1980

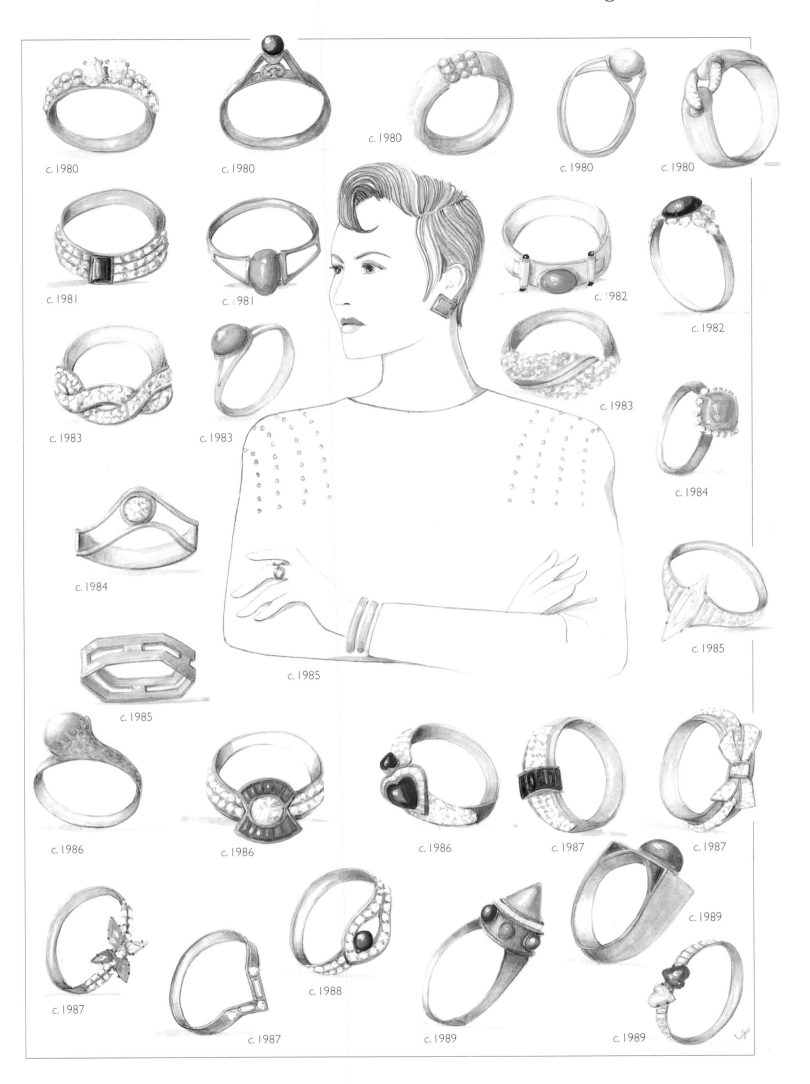

c. 1980

c. 1980

c. 1980

c. 1980

c. 1980

c. 1981

c. 1981

c. 1982

c. 1982

c. 1983

c. 1983

c. 1983

c. 1984

c. 1984

c. 1985

c. 1985

c. 1985

c. 1986

c. 1986

c. 1986

c. 1987

c. 1987

c. 1989

c. 1987

c. 1987

c. 1988

c. 1989

c. 1989

c. 1989

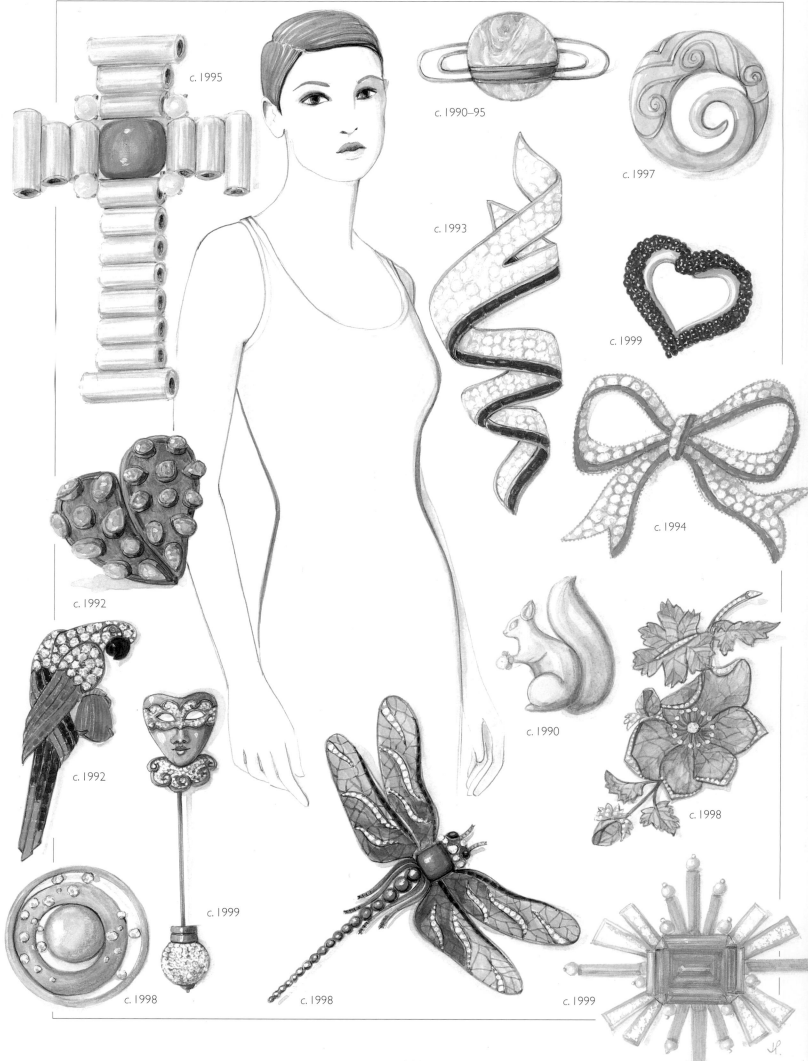

c. 1995

c. 1990–95

c. 1997

c. 1993

c. 1999

c. 1994

c. 1992

c. 1990

c. 1992

c. 1998

c. 1999

c. 1998

c. 1998

c. 1999

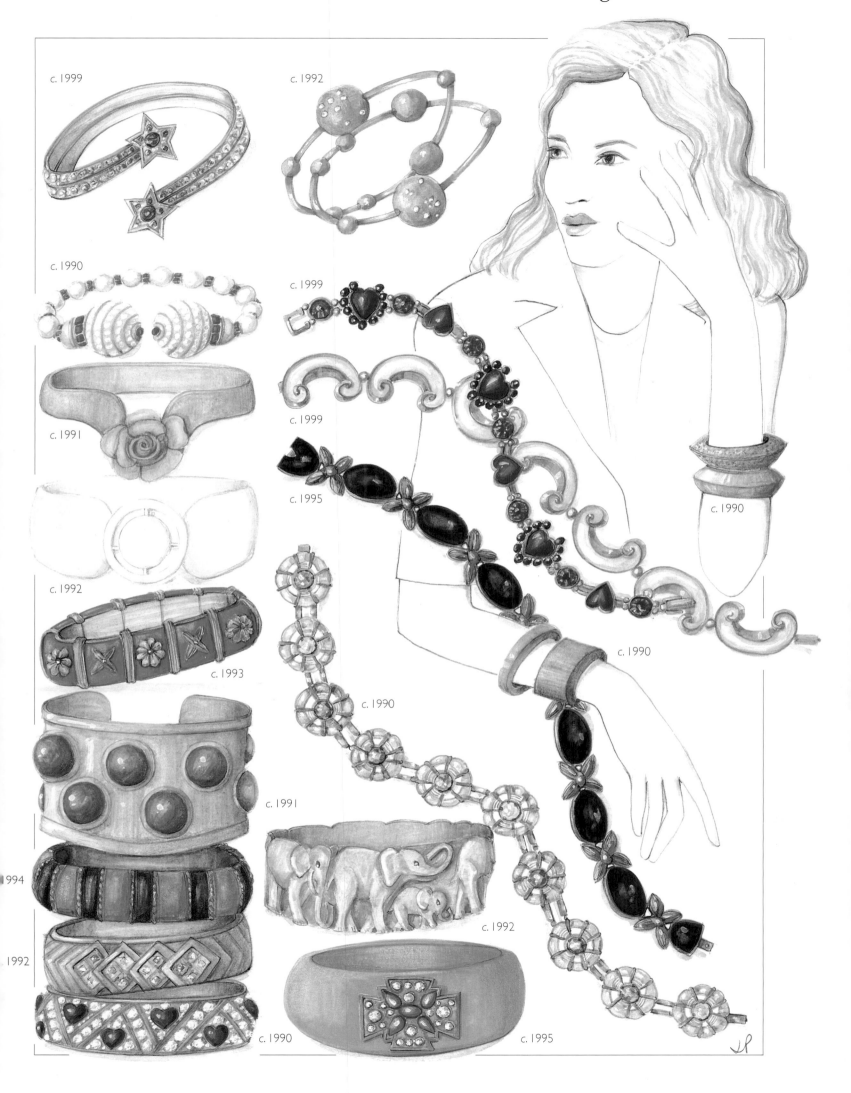

c. 1999

c. 1992

c. 1990

c. 1999

c. 1991

c. 1999

c. 1992

c. 1995

c. 1990

c. 1993

c. 1990

c. 1990

1994

c. 1991

1992

c. 1992

c. 1990

c. 1995

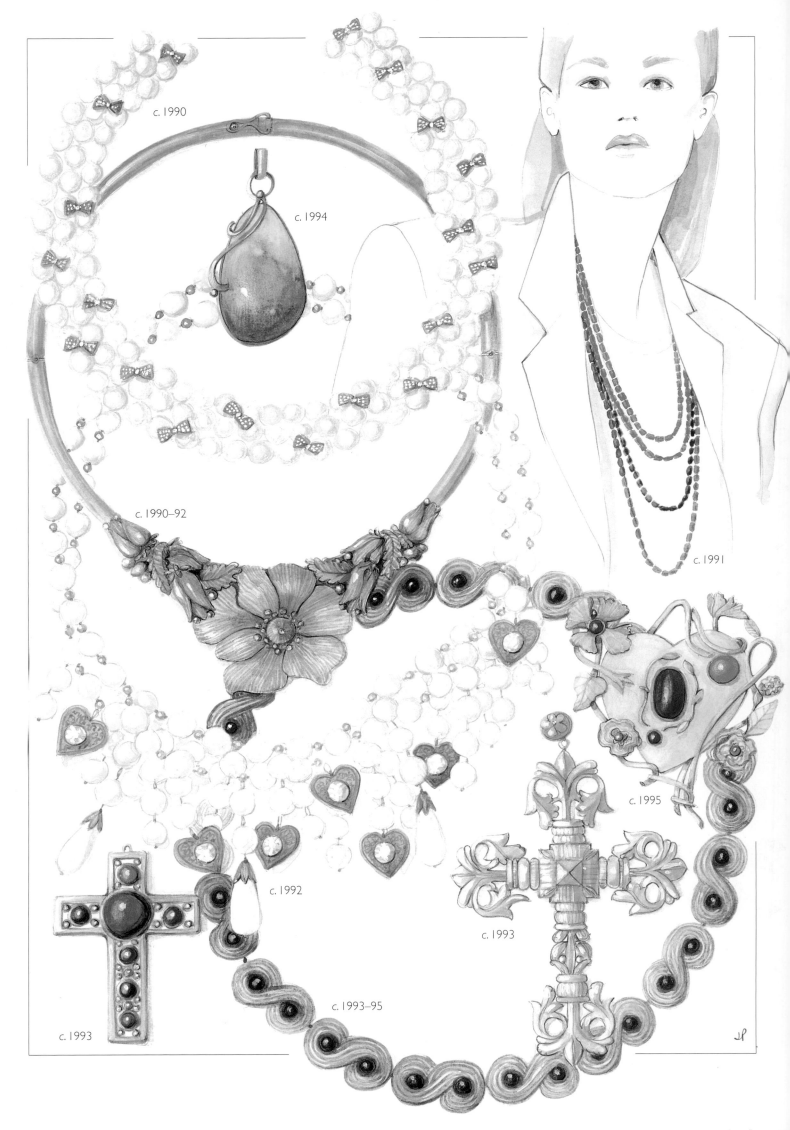

c. 1990

c. 1994

c. 1990–92

c. 1991

c. 1995

c. 1992

c. 1993

c. 1993

c. 1993–95

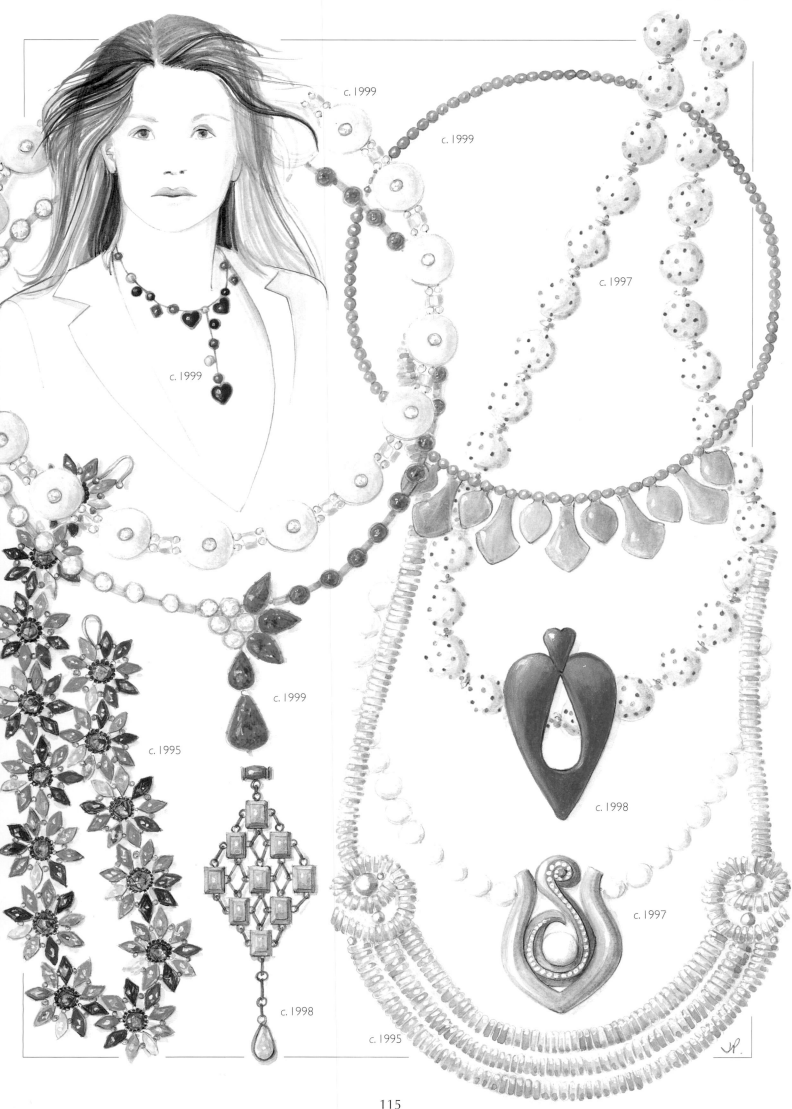

c. 1999

c. 1999

c. 1999

c. 1997

c. 1999

c. 1995

c. 1998

c. 1998

c. 1997

c. 1995

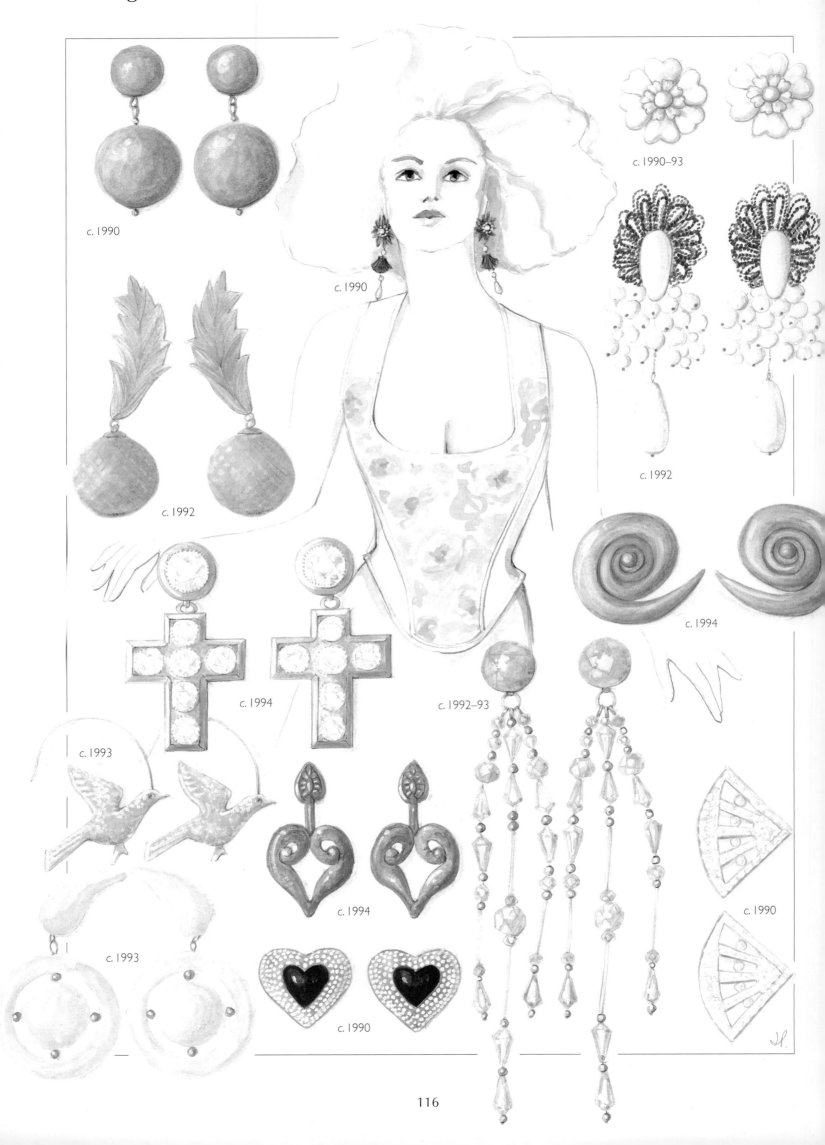

c. 1990

c. 1990–93

c. 1990

c. 1992

c. 1992

c. 1994

c. 1994

c. 1992–93

c. 1993

c. 1994

c. 1993

c. 1994

c. 1990

c. 1990

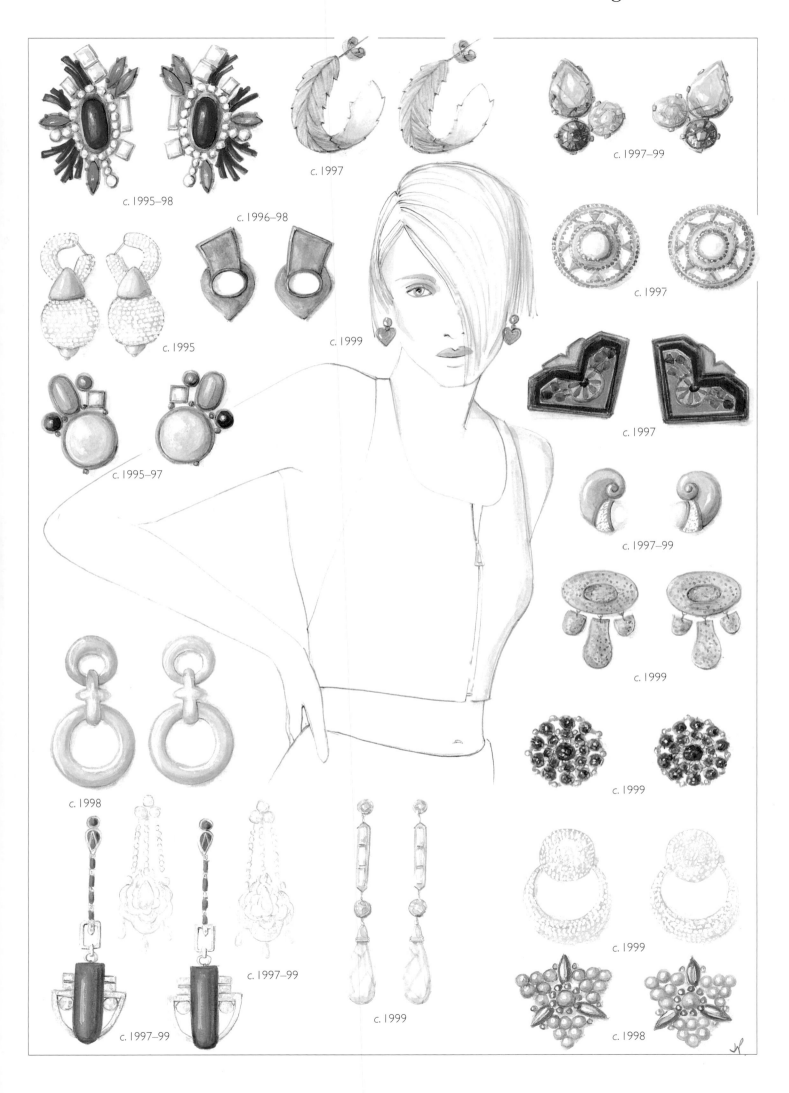

c. 1995–98

c. 1997

c. 1997–99

c. 1996–98

c. 1995

c. 1999

c. 1997

c. 1997

c. 1995–97

c. 1997–99

c. 1999

c. 1998

c. 1999

c. 1997–99

c. 1997–99

c. 1999

c. 1999

c. 1998

Rings 1990–1999

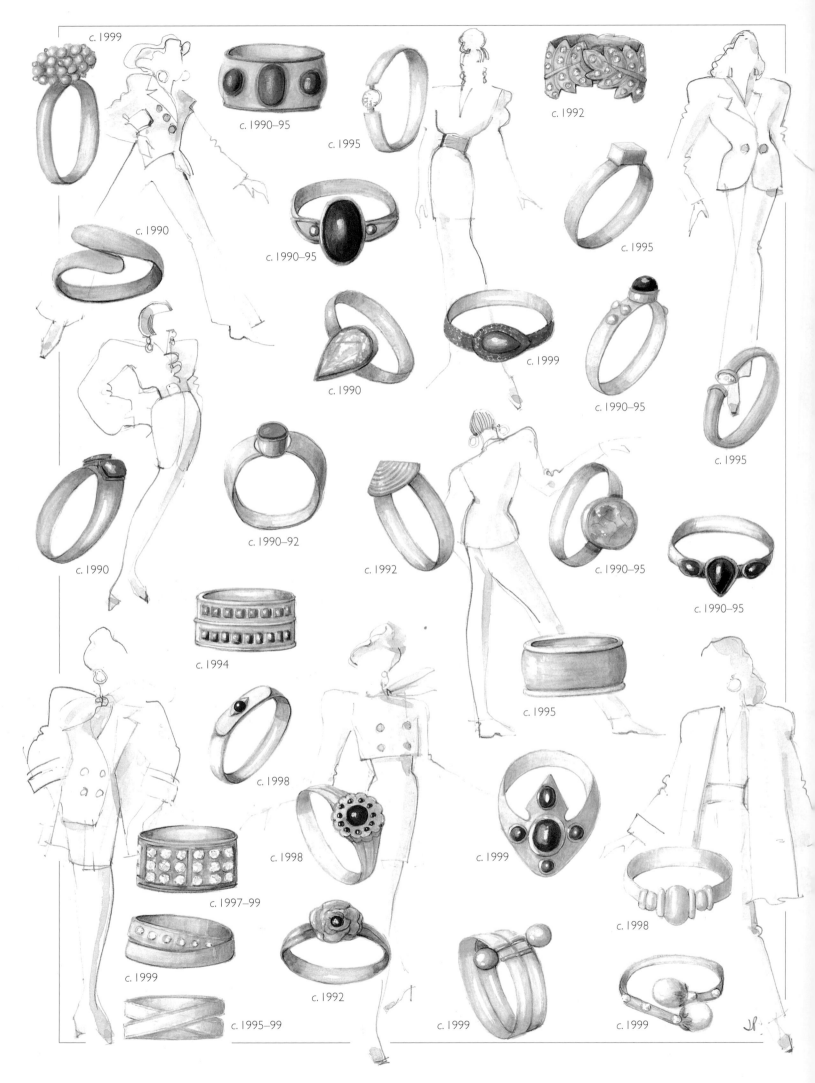

c. 1999

c. 1990–95

c. 1995

c. 1992

c. 1990

c. 1990–95

c. 1995

c. 1990

c. 1999

c. 1990–95

c. 1995

c. 1990–92

c. 1990

c. 1992

c. 1990–95

c. 1990–95

c. 1994

c. 1995

c. 1998

c. 1997–99

c. 1998

c. 1999

c. 1999

c. 1992

c. 1995–99

c. 1999

c. 1999

c. 1998

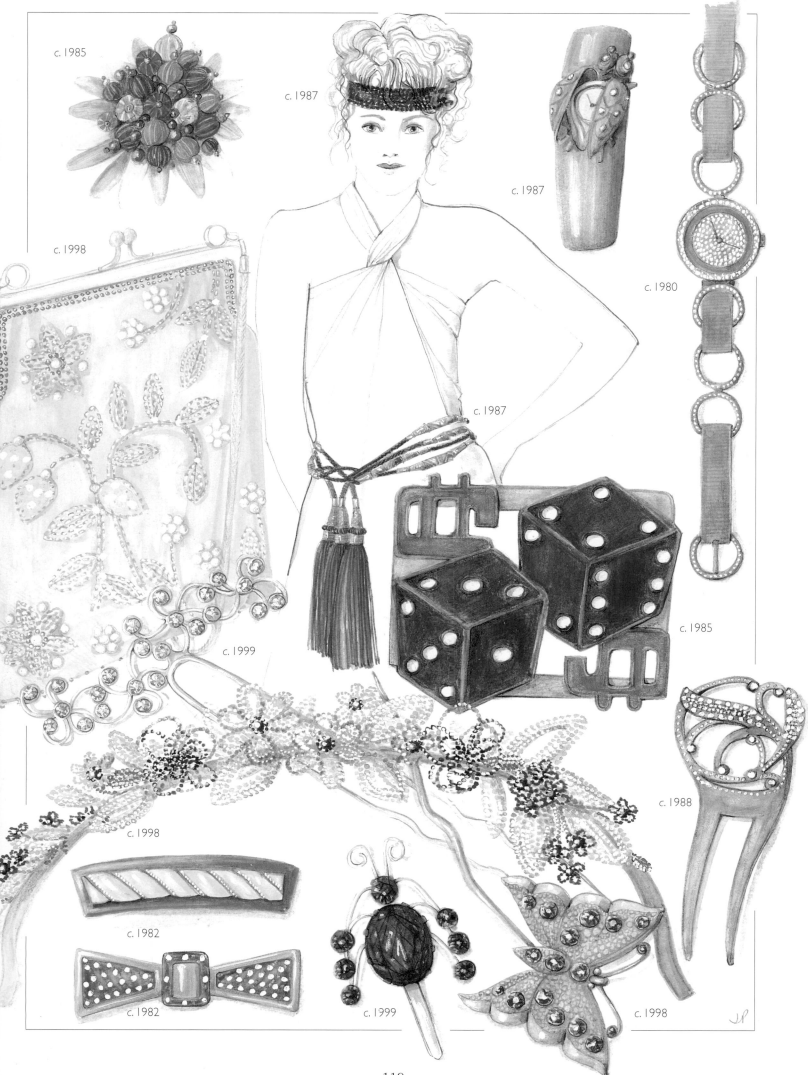

c. 1985

c. 1987

c. 1987

c. 1998

c. 1980

c. 1987

c. 1985

c. 1999

c. 1988

c. 1998

c. 1982

c. 1982

c. 1999

c. 1998

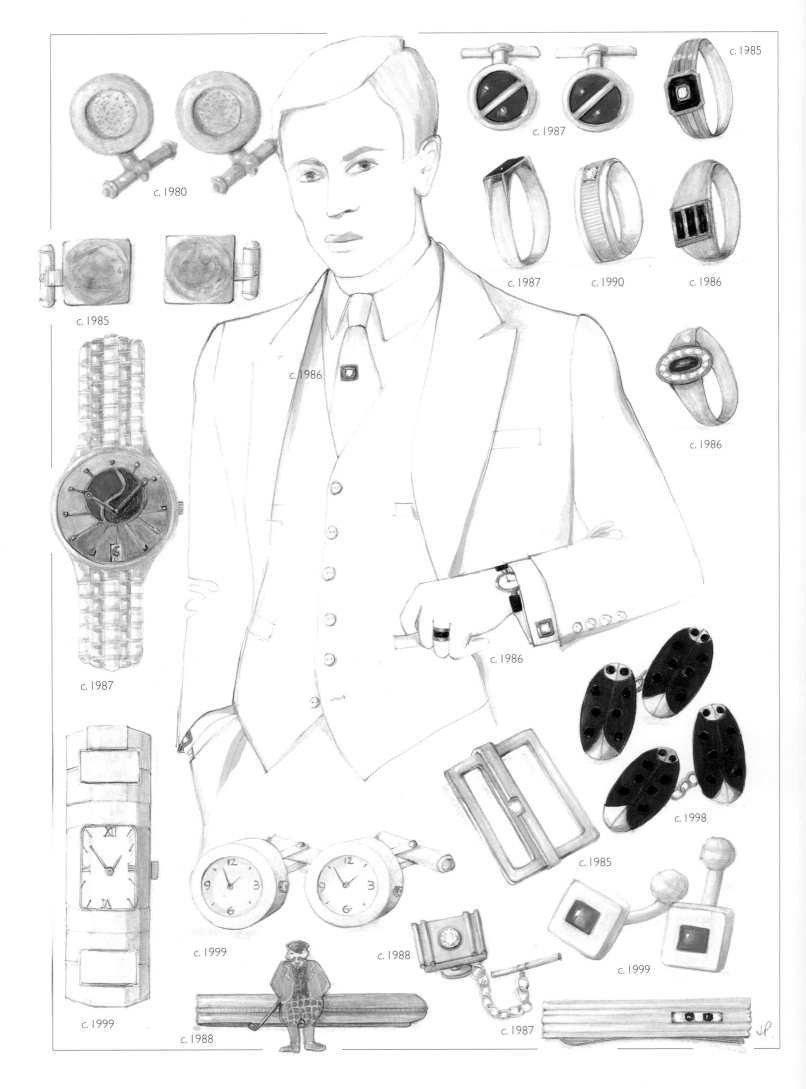

c. 1980

c. 1987

c. 1985

c. 1987

c. 1990

c. 1986

c. 1985

c. 1986

c. 1986

c. 1987

c. 1986

c. 1987

c. 1998

c. 1985

c. 1999

c. 1999

c. 1988

c. 1988

c. 1987

c. 1999

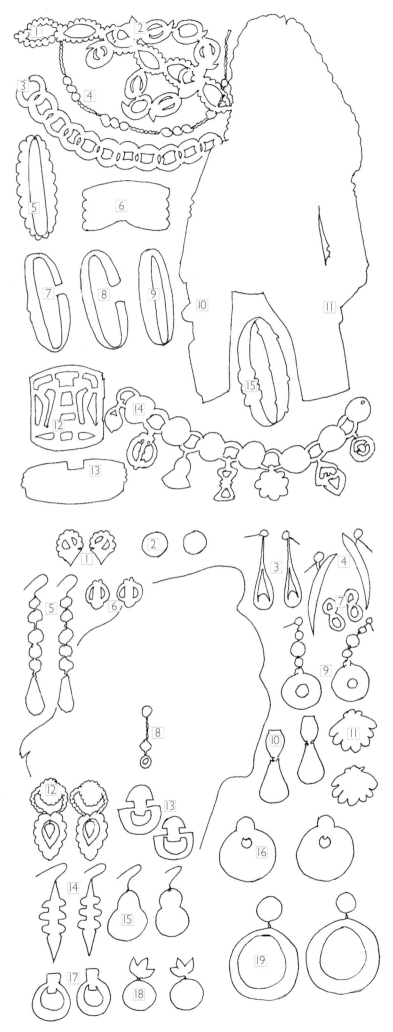

Bracelets and Bangles 1980–1989

1 c. 1980. Gold bracelet, composed of open pointed oval plaques edged with brilliant-cut diamonds, matching two-stone link spacers.
2 c. 1982. Gold bracelet, composed of open wrapover plaques with diamond surround, alternately centrally set with a large cabochon ruby.
3 c. 1981. Gold chain-link bracelet, set with coloured cabochon stones.
4 c. 1981. Delicate bracelet composed of dyed cultured pearls linked by rows of tiny seed pearls and gold wire. 5 c. 1980–84. Gold-coloured metal solid bangle set with coloured-glass beads on outer rim.
6 c. 1980–84. Gold-coloured plastic bangle, swathed design, opening under front wrapover. 7 c. 1987–89. Two-colour gold bangle, overlapping twisted design, open back. In the style of Mappin & Webb.
8 c. 1985. Plastic bangle, set with multicoloured stones in floral design, open back. 9 c. 1980–82. Solid bangle, outer surface decorated with coloured enamel and edged with polished brass, copper interior.
10 c. 1980. Deep hollow copper bangle, beaten design, hinged sides.
11 c. 1980. Deep hollow copper bangle, beaten design, central seam emphasized with polished brass. 12 c. 1985. Gold-coloured polished-metal bangle, abstract open design, textured interior, side hinges.
13 c. 1987–89. Gold-coloured metal bangle, decorated with polished-silver bows, open back. 14 c. 1989. Two-gold charm bracelet composed of flat discs linked with chains, suspended charms include key, bow and linked hearts. 15 c. 1985–89. Gold bangle, twisted vine motif, central opening under flower, the whole set with diamonds.

Earrings 1980–1984

1 c. 1980. Gold clip-on earrings, pierced design set with diamonds.
2 c. 1980. Gold clip-on earrings, set with single central cabochon emerald with diamond surround. 3 c. 1980–84. Gold pendant earrings, single pearl set into pierced drop. 4 c. 1980–84. Sleek feather-shaped gold pendant earrings. 5 c. 1981. Faceted glass-bead pendant earrings, graded colours. 6 c. 1980. Gold-coloured metal clip-on earrings, pierced design set with single semi-precious stone. 7 c. 1982. Gold clip-on earrings, figure-of-eight design set with diamonds.
8 c. 1980–84. Pendant earrings composed of gold-coloured and coloured-glass beads. 9 c. 1981–84. Gold-coloured metal pendant earrings, ethnic design, large engraved discs with pierced centres suspended from line of similar smaller discs. 10 c. 1981. Gold-coloured plastic earrings, engraved onion-shaped pendants set with rows of clear faceted stones, suspended under smaller matching clips. 11 c. 1984. Fan-shaped, clip-on earrings, gold-coloured metal set with clear stones surrounding outsized fake pearl. 12 c. 1981–84. Gold-coloured plastic earrings, ridged pear-shaped pierced pendants, bead inner pendants, clips set with clear stones. 13 c. 1981–84. Gold-coloured metal earrings, half-circle pendants set with rows of clear stones, matching clips.
14 c. 1982. Transparent coloured-glass pendants threaded with matching beads, suspended from gold fixings. 15 c. 1984. Three-colour plastic disc pendants, suspended from gold fixings. 16 c. 1984. Outsized silver-coloured metal disc pendants suspended from matching clips. 17 c. 1983. Graded pendant hoops bound with gold wire, clips set with clear stones. 18 c. 1983. Outsized fake-pearl drops, leaf-design clips set with clear stones. 19 c. 1984. White plastic graded hoops, gold-painted geometric design, matching clips with similar design.

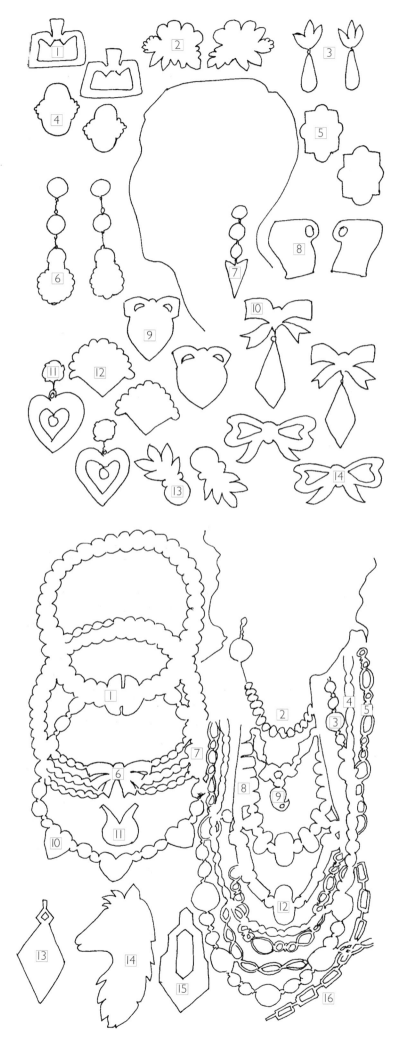

Earrings 1985–1989

1 c. 1985. Gold-coloured metal clip-on earrings, open square hoops below. 2 c. 1985. Frosted-plastic clip-on floral-spray earrings in pastel colours. 3 c. 1985. Gold-coloured metal earrings, three hollow leaf shapes with long fake-pearl pendant drop below. 4 c. 1987–89. Dull gold-coloured metal clip-on earrings, snail-shell design. 5 c. 1987–89. Outsized gold-coloured plastic clip-on earrings, plaque design set with multicoloured plastic stones. 6 c. 1988. Clip-on pendant earrings, composed of three large fake pearls connected by gold wire fixings, end pearl capped with outsized gold-coloured bead covered with smaller beads. 7 c. 1989. Pendant earrings, composed of large black plastic half-bead clips, matching full bead under middle bead covered with faceted clear glass stones, gold-coloured plastic arrow tip. 8 c. 1987. Beaten-silver scroll-design clip-on earrings. 9 c. 1987. Outsized heart-shaped clip-on plastic earrings, decorated with polished-metal looped bow. 10 c. 1986. Outsized gold-coloured metal looped bows, knots set with faceted crystal stone, matching large pointed pear-shaped drops. 11 c. 1988. Clip-on earrings, composed of gold-coloured plastic pierced heart-shaped pendant, faceted coloured stone suspended in centre, matching stone above cup. 12 c. 1988. Square clip-on earrings, enamelled decoration, fan-shaped pearlized-plastic flower trim. 13 c. 1986. Outsized fake-pearl clip-on earrings with tail of multicoloured faceted glass stones. 14 c. 1987. Textured gold-coloured metal clip-on earrings, bow-loop design. In the style of Yves Saint Laurent.

Necklaces and Pendants 1980–1984

1 c. 1980. Short choker necklace, composed of two rows of large pearls, front fastening clasp set with cabochon rubies surrounded by diamonds, gold setting. 2 c. 1982. Short necklace, coloured oval stone beads with gold-coloured metal bead spacers. 3 c. 1982. Long carved ivory-look plastic-bead necklace, three sizes of bead. 4 c. 1982. Long amber-coloured bead necklace. 5 c. 1981. Long gold figure-of-eight linked-chain necklace. 6 c. 1984. Necklace composed of three rows of dyed cultured pearls, front fastening under enamelled looped bow clasp. 7 c. 1980. Long yellow-gold linked-chain necklace. 8 c. 1980. Long ethnic-style necklace, composed of outsized plastic beads spaced with flat circles of coloured felt and with small engraved gold-coloured metal beads at the front, back cord fastening. 9 c. 1981. Ethnic-style necklace, composed of various sized ceramic beads, large amber beads and gold-coloured metal spacers and matching pendant, hook and bead fastening. 10 c. 1982. Short necklace composed of large fake pearls spaced with tiny gold-coloured beads, matching the front larger engraved beads and three heart-shaped motifs, back fastening. 11 c. 1981. Engraved gold-coloured pendant set with fake diamonds. In the style of Monet. 12 c. 1981. Long ethnic-style necklace, composed of patterned ceramic, semi-precious and amber beads. 13 c. 1980. Diamond-shaped engraved gold-coloured metal pendant, set with faceted stones. In the style of Vendôme. 14 c. 1984. Gold pendant, horse-head design, engraved mane set with sprays of diamonds, matching fringe and eye. 15 c. 1980. 1930s-inspired polished gold-coloured metal pendant set with faceted stones. In the style of Vendôme. 16 c. 1984. Textured yellow-gold flat rectangular linked necklace.

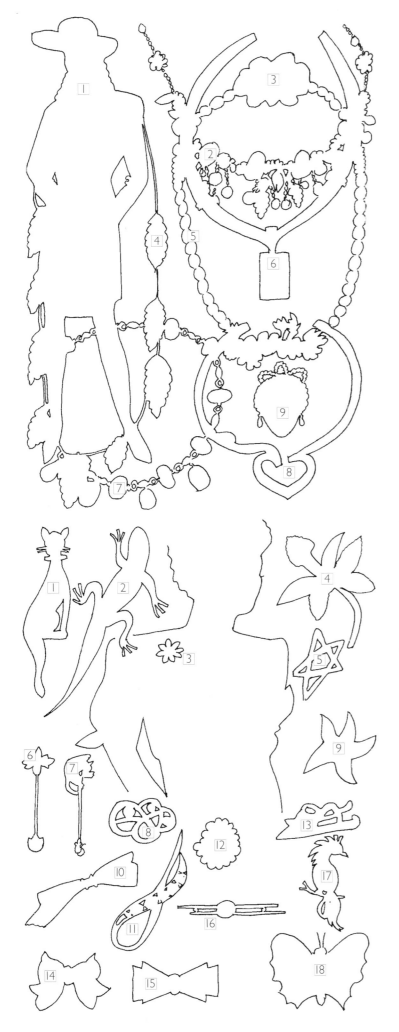

Necklaces and Pendants 1985–1989

1 *c.* 1988. Choker necklace composed of two rows of outsized fake pearls, spaced with diamond-shaped gold-coloured plastic plaques set with small faceted clear stones, back fastening. 2 *c.* 1985. Short necklace composed of large transparent ridged frosted-glass beads, spaced with moulded coloured-glass flowers and leaves, multicoloured glass bead pendants and bunches of frosted coloured-glass grapes, fine bead back with hook fastening. 3 *c.* 1989. Silver floral pendant, enamelled in three colours, edged and decorated with polished silver. 4 *c.* 1987–89. Long necklace composed of various-sized pressed gilded-metal leaves threaded onto fine gold wire cord. 5 *c.* 1988–89. Dull gilded-metal floral-spray pendant, set with tiny fake pearls and faceted clear stones, suspended from long strand of large fake pearls, back fastening. 6 *c.* 1987–89. Rigid silver choker necklace, graded shape at front, open at back, large oblong pendant set with moonstone. 7 *c.* 1985–87. Short gold necklace, composed of oval cabochon turquoise plaques set with two brilliant-cut diamonds, gold chain links spaced with small cabochon emeralds from which are suspended large cabochon turquoise plaques. 8 *c.* 1987. Moulded mottled-plastic choker necklace, flexible shape, heart-shaped front, open back. 9 *c.* 1987. Ceramic doll's-head pendant, painted face, fake-pearl wig, matching drop earrings, wired glass-bead hair ornament.

Brooches, Clips and Pins 1980–1989

1 *c.* 1984–86. Large cat brooch, body and head composed of clear faceted paste stones, coloured eyes, nose and collar. In the style of Butler & Wilson. 2 *c.* 1985. Large lizard brooch, composed of coloured-glass stones. In the style of Butler & Wilson. 3 *c.* 1982. Large floral brooch, textured-gold petals surrounding polished stamens. 4 *c.* 1985–89. Fine beaten-silver floral brooch. 5 *c.* 1988. Polished-gold brooch, open interlinked triangles to form star-shaped design. 6 *c.* 1980. Traditional design gold stickpin and endstop, set with tiny diamonds. 7 *c.* 1988. Gold stickpin, cat-design top with paws and tail set with diamonds, emerald eyes, mouse-design endstop, long curled tail, diamond eyes. 8 *c.* 1980–84. Gold pierced scroll-design brooch set with diamonds and three large cabochon stones. 9 *c.* 1987–89. Plastic starfish brooch, highlighted with gold paint and set with coloured faceted stones. In the style of Billy Boy. 10 *c.* 1987. Tied-bow brooch in polished and textured two-colour golds. 11 *c.* 1980–84. Gold-plated leaf brooch set with large faceted clear stones. In the style of Vendôme. 12 *c.* 1980–84. Large turquoise stone set in gold, asymmetric surround of smaller matching stones and brilliant-cut diamonds. 13 *c.* 1985–87. Triangular enamelled dress clip, edged with gold, topped with large fake baroque pearl under gold-coloured stem and leaves set with clear faceted stones. 14 *c.* 1987–89. Stylized bow brooch set with various-sized diamonds, banded and edged with gold. 15 *c.* 1989. Metal dress clip, stylized bow design enamelled in two colours and edged in gold. 16 *c.* 1987. White and yellow gold bar brooch centrally set with large brilliant-cut diamond. 17 *c.* 1985. Bird brooch, onyx body, marcasite and silver head and plumage. 18 *c.* 1980. Victorian-style butterfly brooch, gold-plated metal, pierced wings and body set with faceted clear-paste stones.

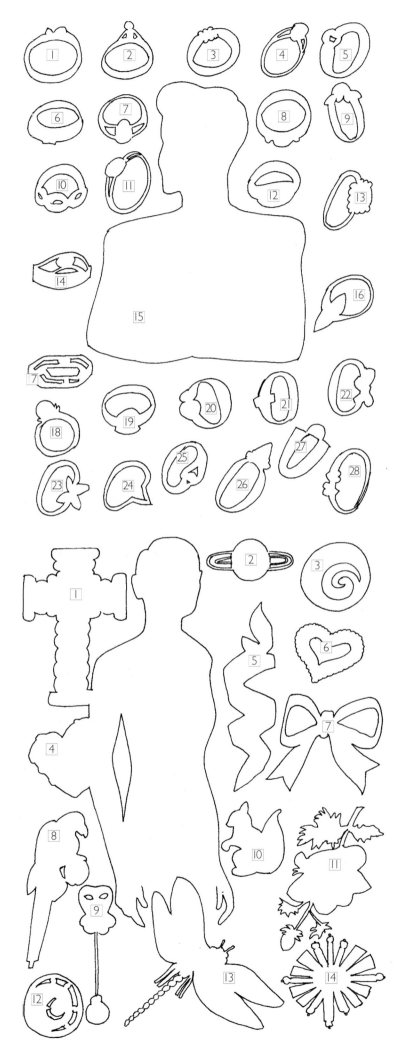

Rings 1980–1989

1 c. 1980. Gold ring set with two pear-shaped diamonds, matching diamond-set shoulders. 2 c. 1980. Gold-plated ring, coloured bead set onto elaborate pyramid. 3 c. 1980. Gold-coloured metal ring, matching central panel of beads. 4 c. 1980. Small baroque pearl set into gold wire ring. 5 c. 1980. Gold ring with split front, joining link set with diamonds. In the style of Chaumet. 6 c. 1981. Gold band, rectangular central coloured stone, shoulders set with clear stones. 7 c. 1981. Gold-coloured metal ring, oval coloured stone set between open shoulders. 8 c. 1982. Gold band, oval cabochon emerald between pillars capped with cabochon rubies. In the style of Bulgari. 9 c. 1982. Gold ring, large ruby with diamond surround. 10 c. 1983. Gold band, linked diamond-set detail across front. 11 c. 1983. Gold-plated ring, cabochon stone between open shoulders. 12 c. 1983. Gold ring, shaped diamond-set front section with gold strap detail. 13 c. 1984. Gold ring, cushion-shaped stone with diamond surround. 14 c. 1984. Large diamond set between parallel asymmetric gold bars, half-band back. 15 c. 1985. Gold ring, linked split front, open shoulders. 16 c. 1985. Gold ring, marquise-shaped diamond between flared diamond-set shoulders. 17 c. 1985. Six-sided gold band, pierced detail. 18 c. 1986. Textured-gold ring, asymmetric claw-set pearl. 19 c. 1986. Gold band, large diamond, emerald fan-shaped panels, diamond-set shoulders. In the style of Mauboussin. 20 c. 1986. Gold ring, large heart-shaped cabochon ruby within diamond frame, small offset cabochon ruby, diamond-set shoulders. In the style of David Morris. 21 c. 1987. Gold band, onyx panel between diamond-set shoulders. 22 c. 1987. Gold band, diamond-set ribbon and bow detail. 23 c. 1987. Gold ring, flower of multicoloured stones, clear stone shoulders. 24 c. 1987. Gold ring, V-shaped front panel set with diamonds. 25 c. 1988. Gold ring, diamond-set wrapover front linked with cabochon ruby button. 26 c. 1989. Gold-coloured metal ring, medieval style, set with semi-precious stones. 27 c. 1989. Gold-coloured band, flat face set with large cabochon stone. 28 c. 1989. Gold ring set with heart-shaped ruby and matching yellow diamond, pavé-set diamond shoulders.

Brooches 1990–1999

1 c. 1995. Outsized cross brooch, composed of sections of tubular metal rods, large central cabochon stone and transparent coloured-glass stones in each corner, can also be worn as a pendant. 2 c. 1990–95. Mother-of-pearl disc brooch set in silver. 3 c. 1997. Coiled matt-gold brooch, raised scroll design. 4 c. 1992. Divided heart-shaped polished-gold brooch, random-set with topaz and peridot. In the style of Solange Azagury-Partridge. 5 c. 1993. Platinum ribbon brooch, set with diamonds, edged on one side with pavé-set rubies. 6 c. 1999. Silver heart-shaped brooch, set with tiny glass beads around open centre. 7 c. 1994. Gold-plated bow brooch, set with faceted clear-paste stones, edged with pavé-set emerald-coloured paste stones. 8 c. 1992. Gold parrot brooch, set with diamonds, emeralds, sapphires and rubies. In the style of Cartier. 9 c. 1999. Gold mask set with tiny pieces of crystal, matching neck frill and ball endstop on long pin. In the style of Swarovski. 10 c. 1990. Gold squirrel brooch, set with diamonds. In the style of Mappin & Webb. 11 c. 1998. Gold floral spray brooch, coloured enamel with painted gold detail, flower centre and edges of petals set with diamonds. In the style of Moira. 12 c. 1998. Gold-coloured metal brooch, composed of small flat disc surrounded by two larger open and offset discs, set and spaced with faceted clear stones. 13 c. 1998. Large gold dragonfly brooch, enamelled wings with gold painted veins, set with sprays of tiny diamonds, matching diamond-set head, eyes and body set with semi-precious stones. In the style of Moira. 14 c. 1999. Large cross brooch, composed of large faceted coloured-glass central stone, surrounded by marcasite plaques and sprays of ridged tubular beads topped with fake pearls.

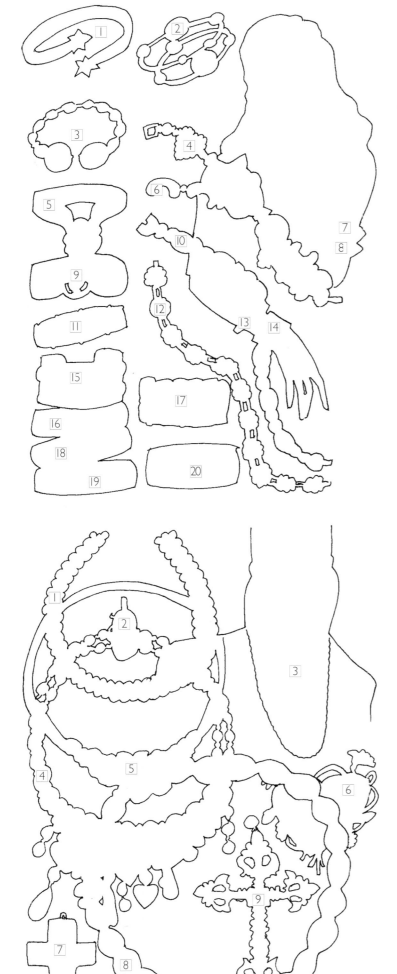

Bracelets and Bangles 1990–1999

1 *c.* 1999. Gold open bangle set with faceted coloured crystal stones, matching star-shaped endstops. 2 *c.* 1992. Two interlocked gold-coloured bangles, threaded with various-sized gold beads, largest beads set with tiny rhinestones. 3 *c.* 1990. Wired fake-pearl open bracelet, coloured-glass bead spacers, endstops set with clear glass beads. 4 *c.* 1999. Gold-coloured bracelet set with heart-shaped coloured crystal motifs. In the style of Angela Hale. 5 *c.* 1991. Gold-coloured plastic bangle, opening concealed under plastic rose set onto shaped front. 6 *c.* 1999. Gold bracelet composed of mother-of-pearl scroll-shaped plaques linked with tiny gold beads. In the style of Angela Cummings. 7 *c.* 1990. Hollow textured gold-coloured metal ethnic-style bangle. 8 *c.* 1990. Hollow polished gold-coloured metal ethnic-style bangle. 9 *c.* 1992. Wide polished-plastic bangle, opening under pierced front disc. 10 *c.* 1995. Bracelet of oval cabochon stones set in gold-plated frames, matching engraved floral spacers. 11 *c.* 1993. Enamelled bangle, decorated with gold-plated motifs, matching lining. In the style of Tiffany & Co. 12 *c.* 1990. Gold-coloured bracelet, pierced floral plaques set with multicoloured crystal stones. 13 *c.* 1990. Narrow gold-plated solid metal bangle. 14 *c.* 1990. Wide gold-plated solid metal bangle. 15 *c.* 1991. Wide gold-coloured plastic bangle, set with large plastic cabochon stones, back open. 16 *c.* 1994. Narrow bangle, raised panels decorated with multicoloured enamels, separated with fine twisted gold wire rope. 17 *c.* 1992. Wide gold bangle, elephant design, emerald eyes. In the style of Cartier. 18 *c.* 1992. Gold-plated bangle, raised geometric design set with faceted multicoloured glass stones. 19 *c.* 1990. Narrow gold bangle set with diamonds and heart-shaped ruby cabochons. In the style of Kutchinsky. 20 *c.* 1995. Wide plastic bangle, front gold-plated cross-shaped plaque set with cabochon stones and fake diamonds.

Necklaces and Pendants 1990–1995

1 *c.* 1990. Short three-strand fake-pearl necklace with scattering of small gold-plated bows each set with tiny crystal stones, back fastening. In the style of David Morris. 2 *c.* 1994. Asymmetrically shaped transparent amber pendant, set in a decorative fine silver mount. 3 *c.* 1991. Long four-strand multicoloured wooden bead necklace. 4 *c.* 1992. Long two-strand fake-pearl necklace, spaced with small gold-coloured beads, matching pendant hearts set with large faceted central stone and caps of long fake-pearl drops arranged among pearl and bead cluster on front of necklace. 5 *c.* 1990–92. Gold-plated rigid choker necklace, large central flower motif with spray of small flower buds, leaves and berries on each side, hinged sides, back opening. In the style of Ilias Lalaounis. 6 *c.* 1995. Gold-plated heart-shaped pendant set with multicoloured glass cabochon stones, wreathed with vine of stylized flowers and leaves, mirror back to pendant. In the style of Christian Lacroix. 7 *c.* 1993. Large gold-plated Byzantine-style cross pendant, pierced background set with multicoloured precious and semi-precious cabochon stones. 8 *c.* 1993–95. Short copper necklace composed of engraved scroll-shaped flat plaques, each set with two ruby-coloured glass cabochon stones, back fastening. 9 *c.* 1993. Large polished-silver cross pendant, medieval-style, with pierced and engraved decoration.

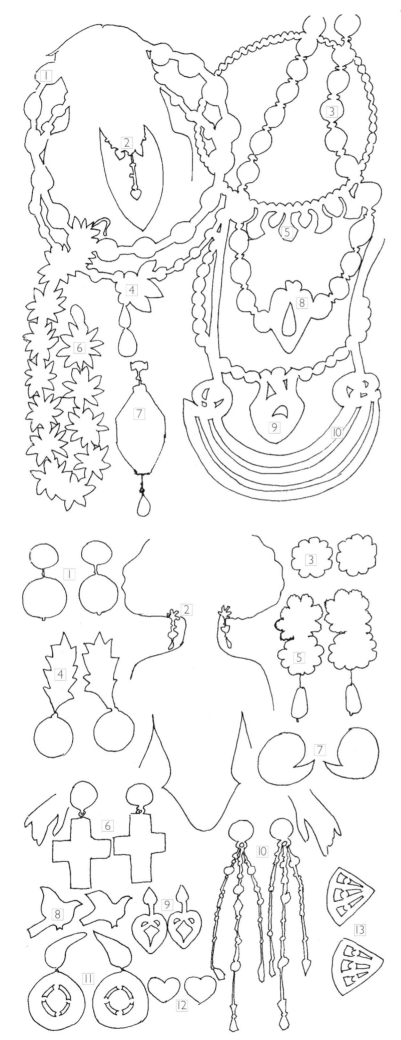

Necklaces and Pendants 1995–1999

1 *c.* 1999. Seventeen mother-of-pearl half beads, each bead set with single clear faceted stone, spaced with matching rectangular stones and fake grey pearls. 2 *c.* 1999. Short gold-plated necklace, plaited chain decorated with multicoloured cabochon stones, matching heart-shaped stones each side and on the base of long central pendant. In the style of Angela Hale. 3 *c.* 1997. Long string of gold-coloured plastic beads, each set with tiny multicoloured faceted stones. 4 *c.* 1999. Short gold-plated necklace, particoloured in clear and emerald-coloured faceted stones, matching asymmetric cluster and pendant. In the style of Green & Frederick. 5 *c.* 1999. Short gold-plated bead necklace, matching fringe of polished cut-out at front. In the style of Agatha. 6 *c.* 1995. Short gold-plated choker necklace, floral design, multi-coloured faceted glass petals and centres. In the style of Butler & Wilson. 7 *c.* 1998. Nine small rectangular gold-coloured metal plaques, each set with single faceted coloured-glass stone, plaques linked with rings and wire to form diamond-shaped pendant, matching pear-shaped drop. 8 *c.* 1998. Polished coloured-plastic heart-shaped pendant with pierced centre. 9 *c.* 1997. Short pearl necklace, gold lyre-shaped central pendant, set with large single pearl, diamond scroll surround. In the style of De Vroomen. 10 *c.* 1995. Long handcrafted strand of gold-painted flat wooden beads matching three rows of beads suspended under decorative scroll support across front.

Earrings 1990–1994

1 *c.* 1990. Gold-coloured polished-plastic clip-on earrings, large ball pendants. 2 *c.* 1990. Shoulder-length gold-plated earrings, floral clips set with large faceted clear stone, surround of similar smaller stones, shell-shaped pendants suspended from fine chain and fake pearls, matching pearl and pear-shaped drops. 3 *c.* 1990–93. Floral pearlized-plastic clip-on earrings, heart-shaped petals, fake-pearl bead centres. 4 *c.* 1992. Leaf-shaped gold-plated clip-on earrings, large faceted coloured-glass ball pendants. 5 *c.* 1992. Pear-shaped fake-pearl clips with surround of wired loops of tiny coloured-glass beads above a cluster of various-sized fake-pearl beads, pear-shaped pendant drops. 6 *c.* 1994. Polished-silver earrings, clips set with a single clear faceted stone, matching stones in outsized cross pendants. 7 *c.* 1994. Outsized coiled gold-coloured polished-plastic clip-on earrings. 8 *c.* 1993. Textured-silver bird earrings, pierced fitting. In the style of Peppi Taylor. 9 *c.* 1994. Textured gold-coloured metal earrings, engraved shield-shaped studs, heart-shaped pendants with pierced centres. 10 *c.* 1992–93. Faceted coloured-plastic clip-on earrings, matching shoulder-length bead pendants. 11 *c.* 1993. Ivory-look leaf-shaped polished-plastic clip-on earrings, matching outsized hoop pendants, pierced centres filled with a flat disc held in position with gold-plated beads. 12 *c.* 1990. Gold-plated heart-shaped clip-on earrings, set with cabochon heart-shaped stone, surrounded by rows of tiny seed pearls. 13 *c.* 1990. Large fan-shaped gilded-metal clip-on earrings, pierced centres edged, lined and decorated with faceted clear-glass stones.

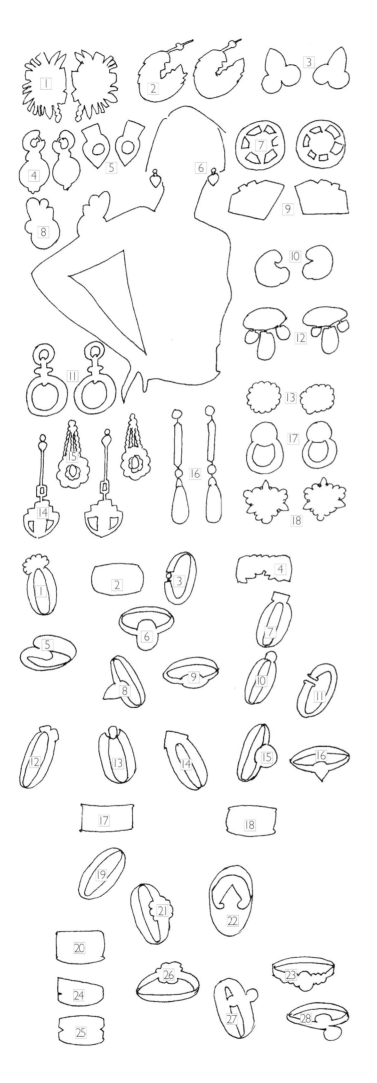

Earrings 1995–1999

1 c. 1995–98. Multicoloured plastic outsized spray-design clip-on earrings. In the style of Christian Lacroix. 2 c. 1997. Gold-plated hoop earrings, engraved curled-leaf design. 3 c. 1997–99. Clip-on earrings, three multicoloured faceted glass stones. In the style of Butler & Wilson. 4 c. 1995. Platinum hoop earrings, set with tiny diamonds, matching ball pendants. 5 c. 1996–98. Tiger's-eye clip-on earrings, framed in gold, pierced centres. 6 c. 1999. Engraved gold-plated clip-on earrings, heart-shaped pendants. 7 c. 1997. Large gold clip-on earrings, pearl bead centres, pierced border. In the style of Ilias Lalaounis. 8 c. 1995–97. Gold clip-on earrings, composed of cluster of various-sized precious and semi-precious cabochon stones. 9 c. 1997. Fan-shaped clip-on earrings, decorated with Egyptian-inspired design in multicoloured enamels. In the style of M.Frey Wille. 10 c. 1997–99. Matt-gold shell-shaped clip-on earrings, set with large pearl and diamond collar. 11 c. 1998. Polished-silver clip-on earrings, pierced centres, matching large pendant hoops. 12 c. 1999. Textured gold-plated clip-on earrings, three matching pendants. In the style of Agatha. 13 c. 1999. 1950s-style clip-on multicoloured faceted glass bead-cluster earrings. In the style of Angela Hale. 14 c. 1997–99. Art Deco-style pendant earrings, set with jade-coloured plastic stones and marcasites. 15 c. 1997–99. Platinum Art Deco-style pendant earrings, set with diamonds. In the style of Moira. 16 c. 1999. Silver pendant earrings, set with faceted semi-precious coloured stones, matching pear-shaped drops. 17 c. 1999. Clip-on earrings, large stud set with tiny clear stones, matching pierced pendant drops. In the style of Green & Frederick. 18 c. 1999. Triangular multicoloured bead cluster clip-on earrings.

Rings 1990–1999

1 c. 1993. Gold bead cluster ring. 2 c. 1990–95. Wide gold band set with three coloured cabochon stones. 3 c. 1995. Gold ring, centre-split set with single diamond. 4 c. 1992. Foliate-design gold band set with small diamonds. 5 c. 1990. Split wrapover design. 6 c. 1990–95. Gold ring set with large cabochon stone, shoulder decorated with beads and wire. 7 c. 1995. Gold ring, cube decoration on front. 8 c. 1990. Gold-plated ring set with pear-shaped faceted coloured-glass stone. 9 c. 1999. Gold-plated ring set with side-on pear-shaped cabochon stone, matching faceted stone surround. 10 c. 1990–95. Silver ring set with semi-precious cabochon stone, shoulders decorated with silver half-beads. 11 c. 1995. Gold ring, one edge of split front set with single diamond, white gold cuffs. 12 c. 1990. Gold-plated ring set with two coloured cabochon stones. 13 c. 1990–92. Gold band, split front with cabochon sapphire. 14 c. 1992. Gold-plated ring, ridged cone decoration on front. 15 c. 1990–95. Gold-plated ring set with large semi-precious cabochon stone. 16 c. 1990–95. Gold ring set with three pear-shaped semi-precious stones. 17 c. 1994. Wide gold band, set with row of sapphires and row of aquamarines. 18 c. 1995. Wide gold band edged with white gold. 19 c. 1998. Gold ring, white gold front plate set with small cabochon ruby. 20 c. 1997–99. Wide gold band, divided into five sections, each set with nine diamonds. 21 c. 1998. Silver-plated ring, floral design, set with central cabochon stone, matching surround of smaller stones. 22 c. 1999. Shield-shaped silver ring set with cabochon stones. 23 c. 1998. Silver ring, bead-design front. 24 c. 1999. Coiled wraparound gold ring, set with row of diamonds. 25 c. 1995–99. Double crossover silver ring. 26 c. 1992. Gold ring, floral design with cabochon ruby centre. 27 c. 1999. Two-tier, two-gold ring, set with a ternate gold bead top and bottom. 28 c. 1999. Gold ring, split crossover front, large pearl endstops, diamond-set shoulders.

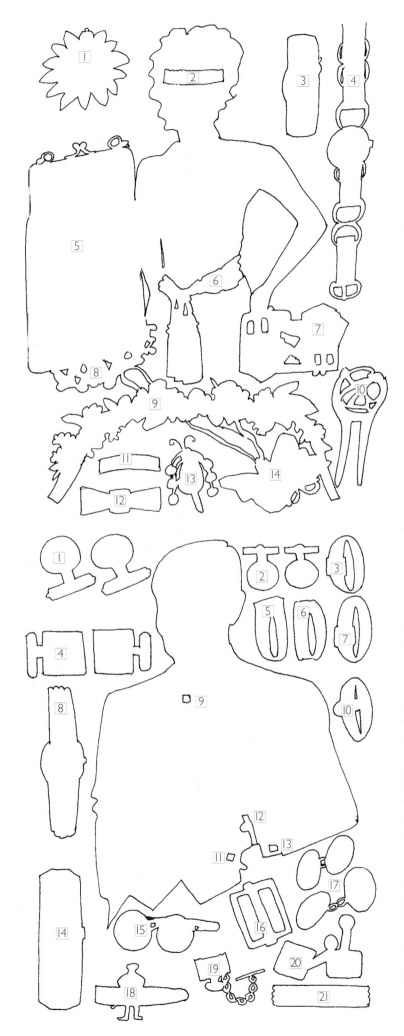

Miscellaneous Jewelry and Jewelled Pieces 1980–1999

1 c. 1985. Summer shoe decoration, wreath design, leather and bead cluster. 2 c. 1987. Multicoloured plastic bead embroidery on stretch-fabric headband. 3 c. 1987. Gold bangle watch, watch face concealed under wings of beetle set with diamonds. In the style of Garrard. 4 c. 1980. Gold wristwatch set with diamonds, silk petersham-ribbon strap, open gold circle links set with diamonds. In the style of David Morris. 5 c. 1998. Silk evening bag, embroidered with fine glass beads and fake pearls, floral design, silver frame and chain handle. 6 c. 1987. Twisted silk cord belt, gold wire spacer links, matching caps to three long silk tassels. 7 c. 1985. Large brass belt-buckle, lucky-dice design decorated with coloured enamels. 8 c. 1999. Long silver hairpin, scroll-design head set with faceted coloured-glass stones. 9 c. 1998. Gold-coloured plastic headband, decorated with wreath of wired multicoloured glass-bead flowers and leaves. 10 c. 1988. Edwardian-style fake-tortoiseshell haircomb set with faceted clear-glass stones. 11 c. 1982. Two-colour plastic hairslide/barrette, twisted central motif set with tiny diamanté stones and gold wire. 12 c. 1982. Two-colour plastic bow hairslide/barrette set with diamanté stones. 13 c. 1999. Silver beetle hairslide/barrette, large faceted-glass central stone, matching head and feet. In the style of Cherry Chau. 14 c. 1998. Gold-coloured metal butterfly hairpin, textured wings and body set with faceted coloured-glass stones. In the style of Johnny Loves Rosie.

Men's Jewelry 1980–1999

1 c. 1980. Gold flat-disc cufflinks, textured centres, bar links. 2 c. 1987. Gold cufflinks, flat discs decorated with two-colour enamel design, bar links. 3 c. 1985. Two-colour banded gold ring, octagonal onyx face set with single diamond. 4 c. 1985. Large silver cufflinks, square plaques set with round flat semi-precious stones, bar links. 5 c. 1987. Gold ring, raised oblong face set with coloured stone. 6 c. 1990. Ribbed yellow-gold ring set with single diamond, edged with white gold. 7 c. 1986. Gold ring, flat square face inset with stripes of black onyx. 8 c. 1987. Outsized gold watch face decorated with coloured enamels, two-colour gold flexible strap. In the style of Omega. 9 c. 1986. Square gold tie-tack set with single diamond. 10 c. 1986. Gold ring, oval cabochon emerald with diamond surround. 11 c. 1986. Wide gold band, inset band of black onyx. 12 c. 1986. Large gold wristwatch, oval face, no numerals, gold hands, ridged leather strap. In the style of Gucci. 13 c. 1986. Square gold cufflinks, set with single diamond. 14 c. 1999. Platinum wristwatch, oblong face with roman numerals set within matching flexible strap. In the style of Alfred Dunhill. 15 c. 1999. Silver cufflinks, working watches, bar links. 16 c. 1985. Small two-piece gold-plated belt-buckle, set with single diamond. 17 c. 1998. Oval silver cufflinks, decorated with coloured enamels to imitate ladybirds, chain links. 18 c. 1988. Gold-plated tie-clip, multicoloured enamel golfer motif on front. 19 c. 1988. Gold tie-tack, square face set with single diamond, pin and cap fastener, safety chain and bar. 20 c. 1999. Solid silver square cufflinks, set with cabochon stone, bent bar and ball links. 21 c. 1987. Gold tie-clip, ridged bar set with rubies and diamonds on one side.

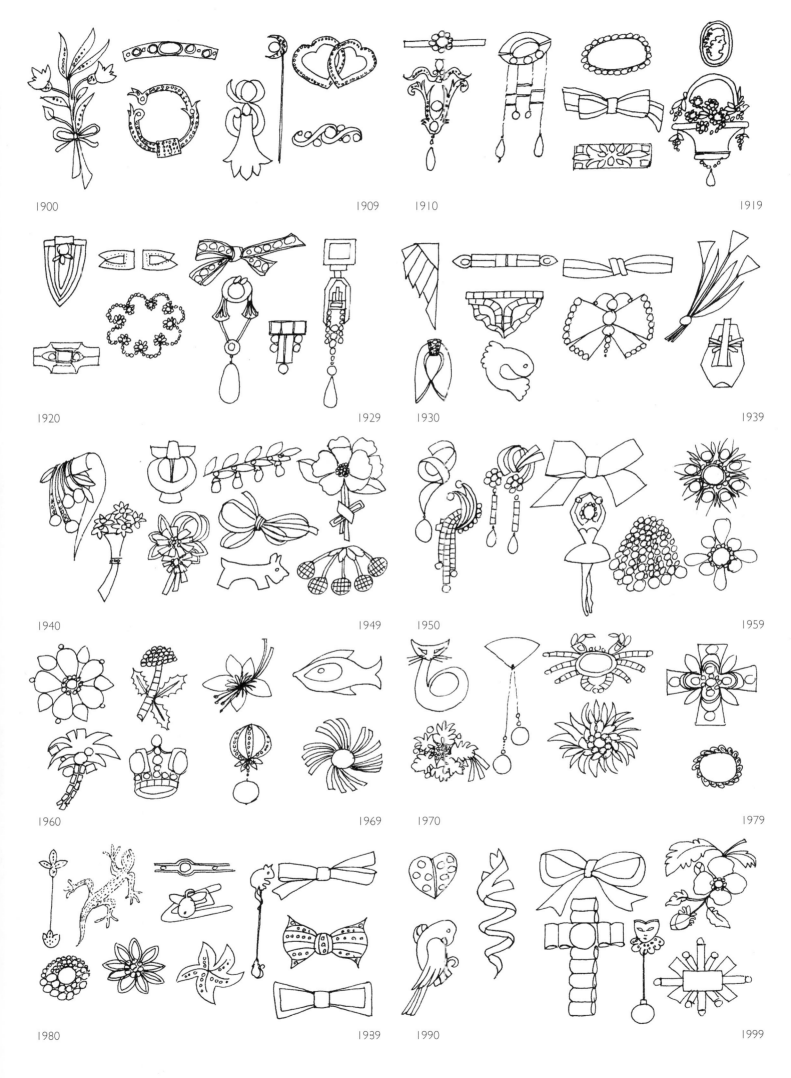

1900   1909   1910   1919

1920   1929   1930   1939

1940   1949   1950   1959

1960   1969   1970   1979

1980   1939   1990   1999

Earrings 1900–1999

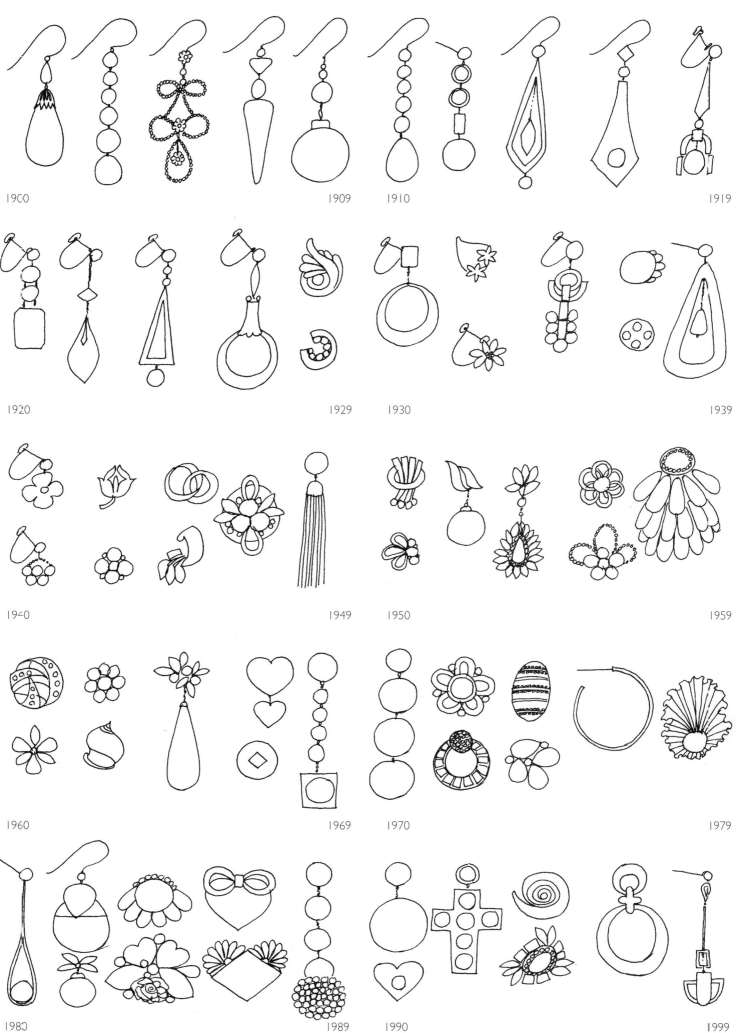

1900

1909 1910

1919

1920 1929 1930

1939

1940 1949 1950

1959

1960 1969 1970

1979

1980 1989 1990

1999

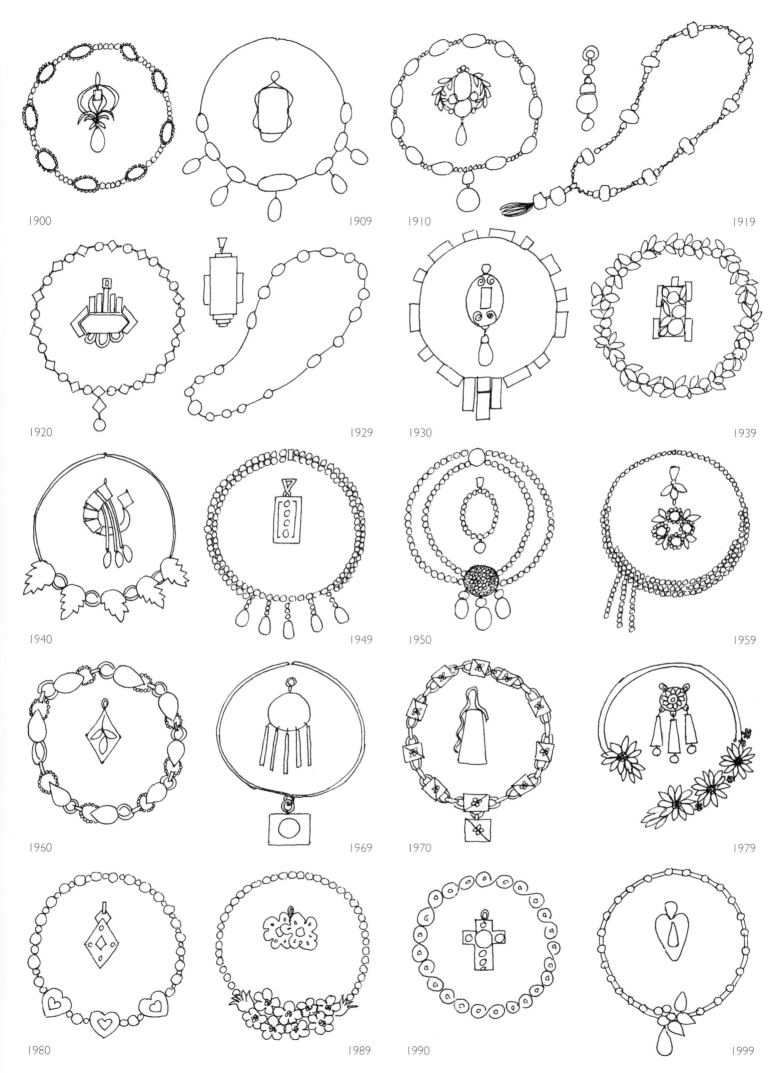

1900

1909

1910

1919

1920

1929

1930

1939

1940

1949

1950

1959

1960

1969

1970

1979

1980

1989

1990

1999

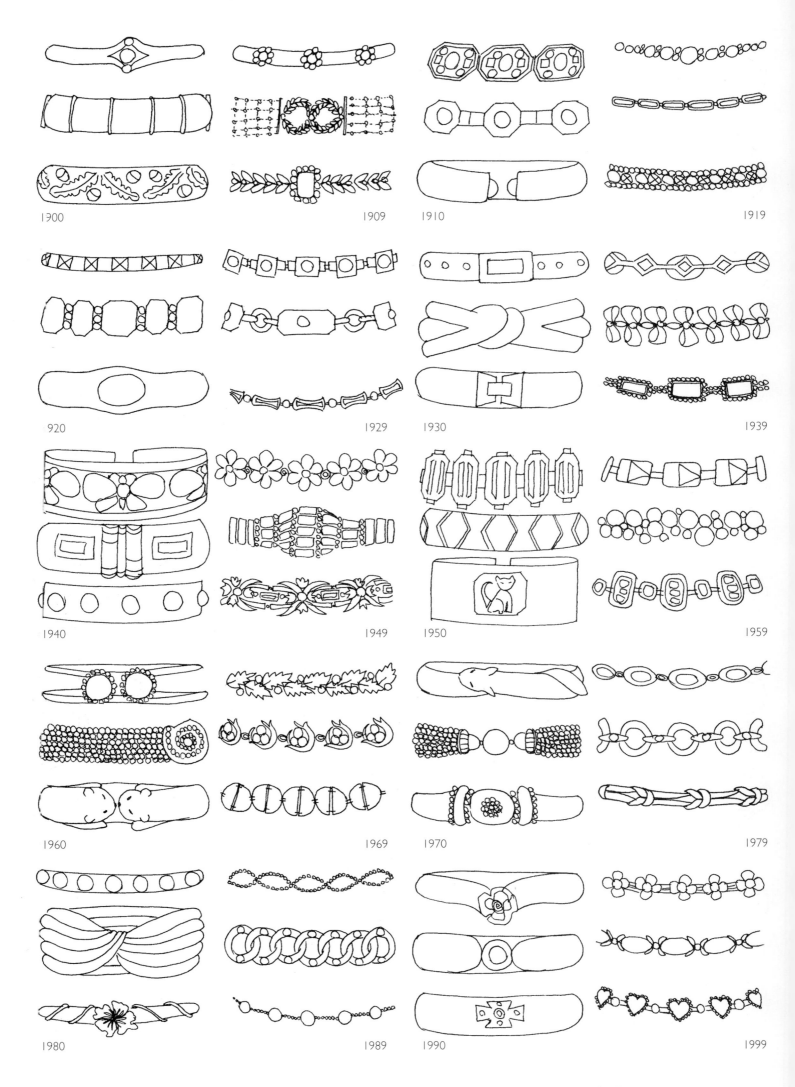

1900

1909

1910

1919

920

1929

1930

1939

1940

1949

1950

1959

1960

1969

1970

1979

1980

1989

1990

1999

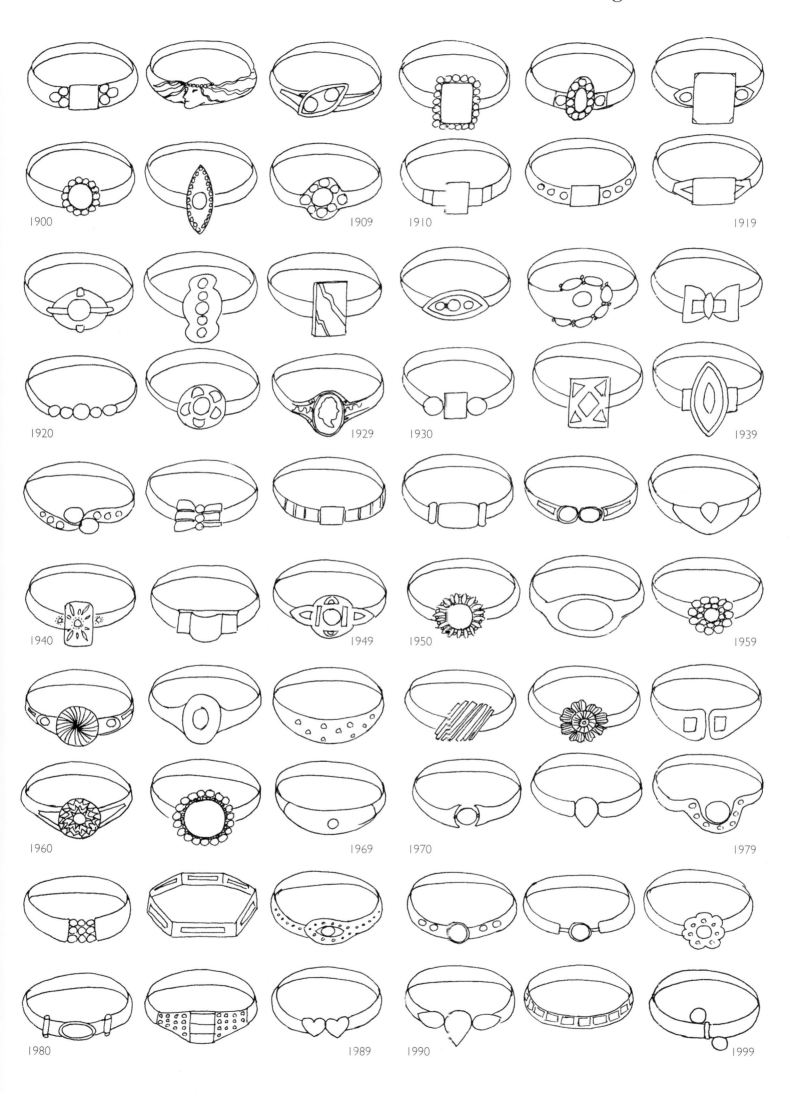

1900

1909

1910

1919

1920

1929

1930

1939

1940

1949

1950

1959

1960

1969

1970

1979

1980

1989

1990

1999

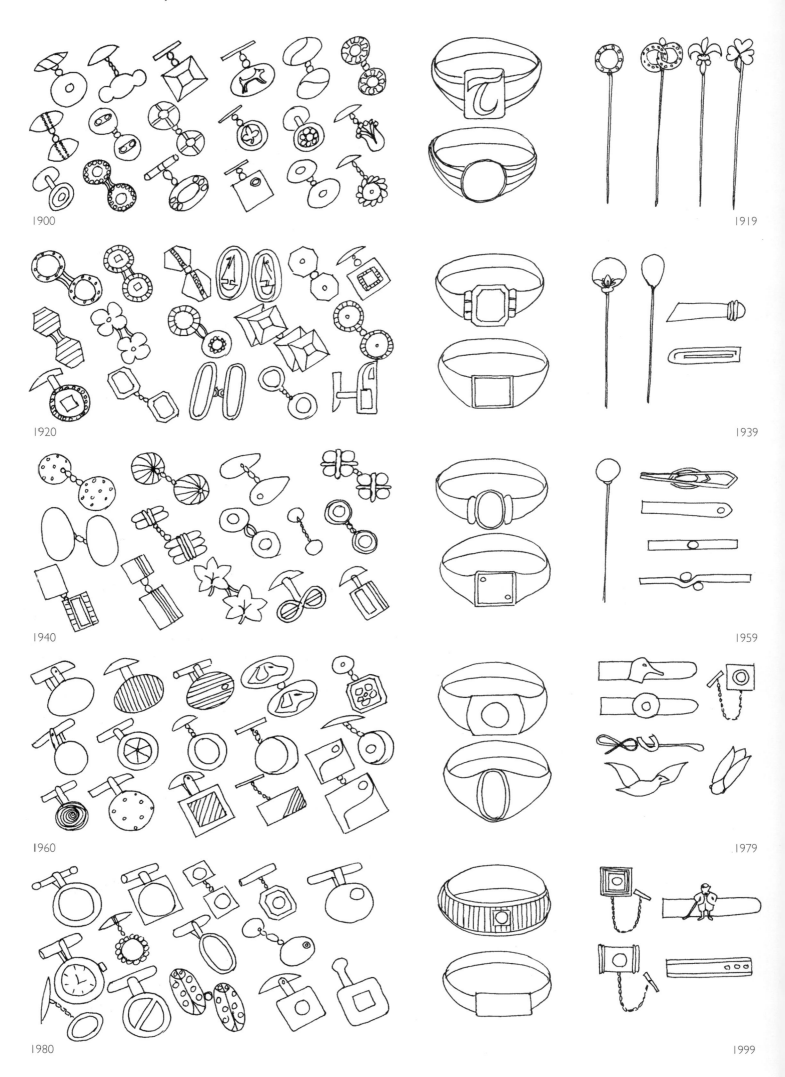

1900

1919

1920

1939

1940

1959

1960

1979

1980

1999

Agatha

Costume jewelry firm founded in Paris in 1974 by Michel Quiniou (b. Mantes-la-Jolie, France; 1947–). The first Agatha boutique opened in Paris in 1976 and as of 2001 the company had 230 boutiques/points of sale in 23 countries. Agatha produces two jewelry collections a year, specializing in fashion-led, upmarket pieces.

Gilbert Albert (1930–)

Born in Geneva, Switzerland. Albert studied at the School of Industrial Arts in Geneva. He was then employed by the jewellers and watchmakers Gallopin & Cie and served as workshop head at Patek Philippe SA before founding his own company in 1962. The company is known for abstract gold jewelry incorporating unusual materials such as shagreen, peacock feathers, tiger claws, arrow tips and silks.

Kate Allen (dates unknown)

British-born designer of pieces in the Arts and Crafts style, including belt-buckles and clasps inspired by Celtic patterns. Active in the early years of the twentieth century.

Artwear *see* Robert Lee Morris

Charles Robert Ashbee (1863–1942)

Born in Middlesex, UK. An architect, designer, writer and social reformer, C. R. Ashbee was also a self-taught silversmith and jeweller who became one of the most important figures in the promotion of the Art Nouveau style. In 1888 he founded the Guild and School of Handicraft in London and in the 1890s began designing jewelry in simple forms, made from silver wire and inexpensive coloured stones such as turquoise, moonstone and opal. He was instrumental in the development of jewelry for *Liberty & Co. He is famous for his interpretations of the peacock motif and also for his stylized natural motifs, especially leaves and petals.

Asprey & Co.

Asprey & Co. was founded in 1781 in Mitcham, Surrey, UK, by William Asprey. William's son and grandson, both named Charles, developed the business. After entering a partnership with a stationer in 1841, the firm moved to Bond Street in 1847. Asprey flourished in the nineteenth century as a supplier of luxury goods and was granted two royal warrants. The jewelry department houses an extensive collection of rare stones and provides services such as the re-setting of family heirlooms and the creation of one-off pieces. Asprey supplied Madonna with her wedding tiara – a piece dating from circa 1910 made up of 767 diamonds. The firm also created a costume jewelry version of the 'Titanic Diamond' for Kate Winslet to wear in the film *Titanic*. In 1998 Asprey merged with *Garrard & Co., but the two companies separated in 2001.

Solange Azagury-Partridge (1961–)

Born in London, UK. After taking a degree in French and Spanish, Azagury-Partridge worked for one year for *Butler & Wilson. She then moved to the twentieth-century art and jewelry dealer Gordon Watson. In 1987 she designed her own engagement ring, the success of which encouraged her to set up her jewelry business in London in 1990. She mixes gold and uncut semi-precious and precious stones in sculptural settings.

Mogens Ballin (1871–1914)

Danish artist and designer who established his workshop in 1900. Ballin's jewelry used powerful organic forms in various metals, including silver and pewter, set with semi-precious stones. *See also* Georg Jensen.

Slim Barrett (1960–)

Born in County Galway, Ireland. Barrett studied Fine Art at the Regional Technical College in Galway and arrived in London in 1983, when he began to design jewelry. He has received commissions from Galliano, *Chanel, Ungaro, Versace and Montara, among others. His work is most often described as 'whimsical' and he is credited with starting the 1990s craze for tiaras. His private clients have included the Princess of Wales, Madonna and Cher. He also created a fairytale gold crown studded with diamonds for Victoria Adams ('Posh Spice') for her wedding to David Beckham.

Suzanne Belperron (1899–1983)

French-born Suzanne Belperron studied at the Ecole des Beaux-Arts in Paris. In 1918 she began a decade-long collaboration with the Parisian jeweller René Boivin. In 1933 she began designing for Bernard Herz, an important pearl merchant of the period. During the Second World War Herz was deported and when in 1945 Belperron went into partnership with his son, Jean Herz, the firm became known as Herz-Belperron. Suzanne Belperron's designs are characterized by bold, pure lines, with restrained ornamentation, and with both matt and shiny surfaces. She frequently used precious and semi-precious materials together. Most of her designs were executed by the Paris workshop of Groene et Darde. She continued to design up to her death, but never signed the pieces, arguing that her designs were immediately recognizable.

BillyBoy (1960–)

Born in Vienna, Austria. Influenced by his mother and aunts, all of whom were clients of the great couturiers, BillyBoy started a collection of haute-couture dresses at the age of 13. Aged 15, he founded Surreal Couture, followed five years later by Surreal Bijoux, on the rue de la Paix, Paris. BillyBoy has created 'surrealist' jewels for Thierry Mugler and Charles Jourdan, and counts Lauren Bacall, Elizabeth Taylor and Boy George among his clients. He is also well known for his collection of Barbie dolls.

Bogoff *see* Jewels by Bogoff

Boucher & Cie

Marcel Boucher (born France; d. 1965) trained as an apprentice at *Cartier. He emigrated to the USA in the early 1920s and during the early 1930s designed shoe buckles for Mazer Brothers in New York.

In 1937 he established the Marcel Boucher & Cie Company in New York with a collection of 12 brooches which Saks Fifth Avenue bought and successfully reproduced. Boucher produced exquisite costume jewelry in the classical tradition, using exceptionally high-quality rhinestones.

Boucheron
Jewelry firm established in Paris in 1858 by Frédéric Boucheron (1830–1902), who had trained with the French engraver and chaser Jules Chaise. In the 1860s Boucheron became the first jeweller to establish a workshop on the Place Vendôme, which was to become the worldwide symbol of 'Haute Joaillerie'. Louis Boucheron, Frédéric's son, took over the running of the firm on his father's death. The firm initially achieved fame for its high-quality jewelry inspired by natural forms, but it kept pace with changing fashions and later made excellent pieces in the Art Nouveau and Art Deco styles. Boucheron describes itself as 'the Jeweller of Time': it designed the first jewelry watch bracelets as well as the interchangeable invisible clasp bracelet.

Bulgari
Italian jewelry firm founded by the Greek-born Sotirio Bulgari (1857–1932). A specialist in the art of engraving, Sotirio emigrated to Naples in 1881 and opened his first shop in Rome in 1884. He was later joined in the business by his sons Constantino and Giorgio and in the 1930s turned from engraving to the production of jewelry. Giorgio Bulgari dedicated his life to creating a 'Bulgari style'. This new aesthetic replaced the 'French style' – a diamond or other precious stone set in prongs – with a coloured stone set in a handcrafted gold bezel, in a frame of tapered baguette diamonds, and with the centre encased in a heavy gold chain. Bulgari designs harked back to the Renaissance, to Etruscan art and to Ancient Rome. It was the first firm to use antique coins and handmade gold chains in fine jewelry, and in the 1950s used yellow gold instead of platinum or white gold in the setting of precious stones. It also revived the cabochon cut. Constantino Bulgari wrote *Argentieri, Orafi e Gemmari d'Italia*, the only directory of hallmarks of Italian silver through the ages. Sons and nephews continue the family tradition.

Butler & Wilson
Nicky Butler (b. 1946) and Simon Wilson (b. 1944) started as antique dealers, selling jewelry, particularly from the Art Nouveau and Art Deco periods, in London street markets. Noting the popularity of such jewelry, they began to make copies by hand, before moving into mass production. They set up the company Butler & Wilson in 1968, selling their own line based on reproductions of period styles, including, in the 1980s, a highly successful turn-of-the-century lizard brooch in a variety of colours and designs.

Hattie Carnegie (1886–1956)
Born Henrietta Kanengeiser in Vienna, Austria. Carnegie was primarily a clothes designer: she launched her first clothing

collection in New York in 1918. Famous from the 1930s to the 1950s for her restrained, conventional suits and little black dresses, she also produced quirky, theatrical, colourful costume jewelry, often in matching sets.

Cartier
French jewelry firm, also famous for the development of the wristwatch, established by Louis-François Cartier (1819–1904) in Paris in 1847. The firm quickly prospered with the support of clients such as the Empress Eugénie. Cartier's son Alfred (1841–1925) took over premises at 13 rue de la Paix in 1898, the same year in which Alfred's son Louis (1875–1942), the driving artistic force behind the Cartier style, joined the firm. In 1902 Alfred's second son, Pierre (1878–1964), set up a branch in London and in 1909 the direction of the London branch was given to the youngest family member, Jacques Cartier (1884–1942). The company received the first of many royal warrants in 1904, around which time maharajas and oriental princes began to become ardent admirers of the Cartier style. In 1908 a branch opened in New York. In the early years of the century, Cartier specialized in Belle Epoque diamond dog collars, stomachers, lavallières and tiaras in the 'garland style' set in platinum. After the First World War Louis Cartier began introducing the new lines of Art Deco. He was supported by talented collaborators, among them Charles Jacqueau (1885–1968), Jeanne Toussaint (1887–1978) and Peter Lemarchand (1906–70). In 1933 Toussaint was put in charge of the jewelry and under her direction a highly successful line in yellow- and gold-coloured stones was produced. In 1972 Robert Hocq (d. 1979) became President of Cartier Paris, and two years later Hocq's daughter Nathalie (b. 1951) began to run the high-fashion jewelry department and to promote 'Les Must de Cartier' – a boutique collection which sells jewels at more affordable prices.

Chanel
The jewelry designs of the couturier Coco Chanel (b. Saumur, France; 1883–1971) combine primitivism with sophistication and are characterized by their unusually large size, their uneven shapes, their innovative use of materials and their crude execution. Chanel collaborated with highly talented designers, including Count Etienne de Beaumont, whom she hired in 1924. In 1931 she met the illustrator Paul Iribe (1883–1935) and their designs were seen in 1932 in a hugely successful exhibition of sumptuous diamond and platinum jewelry with delicate settings, based on three themes: bows, comets and feathers. ✳Fulco di Verdura started his jewelry career at Chanel, designing for her from 1927 to 1934 and producing some quintessential Chanel pieces, including a number of variations on the theme of the Maltese cross. Chanel is also known for her famous strings of obviously fake pearls and for precious stones in ornamental settings of Byzantine inspiration. From 1924 on, Chanel's jewelry was often made by ✳Maison Gripoix.

Cherry Chau
Fashion accessories company launched in 1992 by Cherry René-Bazin (b. Hong Kong; 1954–). René-Bazin studied at the London

College of Fashion. The Cherry Chau company specializes in hair accessories, including diamanté clips, beaded combs and tiaras, and jewelry made from semi-precious stones.

Chaumet
Jewelry company first established in Paris in 1780 by Marie-Etienne Nitot. It was famous in the eighteenth and early nineteenth centuries for making pieces for Napoleon, but was not given the name Chaumet until 1907, when Joseph Chaumet joined the firm. He rebelled against the large, overly decorative jewelry of the time, and created refined pieces in the Art Nouveau style. During the twentieth century the company adapted successfully to changing fashions.

Coro
Coro, started in 1929 in Providence, Rhode Island, USA, took its name from the first two letters of the surnames of its founders, Emanuel Cohn and Carl Rosenberger, who had been in business together since 1901. Coro is perhaps the world's largest costume jewelry company. It has used more than fifty different trademarks, the most important of which are Coro, Corocraft and Coro-Duette. The company is best known for its 1940s pieces, such as retro brooches and cuffs, animal and flower brooches, and double clips.

Angela Cummings (1944–)
Born in Austria. Cummings studied goldsmithing, gemmology and jewelry design in Hanau, Germany. She was made assistant to Donald Claflin at *Tiffany & Co. in 1967 and introduced her debut collection six years later. In 1983 she started her own company in Connecticut, USA. Cummings draws inspiration from flora and fauna and is known for jewelry that mixes the organic and the abstract, including pieces that feature diamonds set in exotic species of wood.

Nelson Dawson (1859–1942) and Edith Dawson (1862–1928)
Jewelry designers in the Arts and Crafts style. Their jewels have typical metalwork settings and often incorporate deep-coloured enamels of flowers, birds and insects.

Jean Desprès (1899–1980)
Born in Souvigny-Allier, France. In addition to their famous glass-making company, Desprès's parents had a jewelry business in Paris, to which they sent their son as a young boy to learn the craft. During the First World War Desprès worked on the production of aeroplanes and remained fascinated by the machine-age aesthetic throughout his life. He worked in metal, silver, gold and pewter, and his designs are strongly modernistic, with geometrical patterns and motifs, though in the late 1920s, when he began a collaboration with the Surrealist artist Etienne Cournault, his pieces became less rigid.

De Vroomen Design
Founded in 1976 by Leo de Vroomen (b. near Leiden, Holland; 1941–). De Vroomen trained as a goldsmith in Holland before moving to England in 1965. After several years' lecturing in jewelry design at the Central School of Art and Design in London, he set up a studio/workshop in 1970 with his wife, Ginnie. The company was founded six years later and Gisèle Moore joined as in-house designer in 1982. De Vroomen Design is chiefly known for its bold, innovative jewelry based on two main themes: sensuously sculptured repoussé which celebrates the warmth and malleability of gold, and enamels of every colour which are used to accentuate precious and semi-precious stones.

Jean Dinh Van (1927–)
Born in Boulogne-sur-Seine, France. Son of a Vietnamese father and a French mother, Jean Dinh Van produced his first jewelry under his own name in 1965, after ten years' apprenticeship with Cartier and study at the Ecole des Arts Décoratifs. In 1967 he created a ring for Pierre Cardin and made his debut with a collection for Cartier New York. In 1976 he opened a boutique on the rue de la Paix in Paris. Dinh Van is known for minimalist, 'easy-to-wear' jewelry in stylized, simple forms.

Alfred Dunhill
Established by Alfred Dunhill as Dunhill Motorities in London in 1891, the firm diversified to pipes in 1910 and to luxury accessories, including lighters and pens, in 1924. The firm is also known for its production of watches, from the Dunhill Dashboard Watch of 1895 to the Millennium ranges of wristwatches launched in 1981 and the Dunhillion Watch of 2001.

Erickson Beamon
Costume jewelry house founded in New York in 1983 by Karen Erickson (b. Detroit, USA; date unknown) and Vicki Sarge (b. Detroit, USA; 1954). In 1995 Sarge opened a branch in London. Erickson Beamon jewelry is fashion-led and the company has worked with Alexander McQueen, Julien Macdonald, Dries Van Noten and Anna Sui, among others.

Fabergé
In 1870 Peter Carl Fabergé (1846–1920) took over the firm started by his father, Gustav Fabergé (1814–81), in St Petersburg in 1842. He was later joined by his brother, Agathon, and by his sons, Eugène and Alexander. Fabergé is famous for its innovative creations in gold, enamelling and gemstones, and in particular for the jewelled eggs made from 1884 as Easter gifts from the Tsar to the Tsarina. It created a small range of jewelry, much of it in the Art Nouveau style. The factory closed after the 1918 Revolution.

Theodor Fahrner
Jewelry house, originally founded as Seeger & Fahrner in Pforzheim, Germany, in 1855. Theodor Fahrner took over the sole running of the firm in 1855. After his death in 1919 the company was sold to Gustav Braendle and the firm became known as Gustav Braendle, Theodor Fahrner, Succ. Famous at the turn of the century for its Art Nouveau designs, in the 1920s the company produced quintessential geometric Art Deco jewelry, including some of the finest brooches of the period. From 1952 it was headed by Gustav's son, Herbert Braendle, and was dissolved on his death in 1979.

Gerda Flöckinger (1927–)

Born in Innsbruck, Austria. Flöckinger moved to London in 1938. She studied Fine Arts at St Martin's School of Art, and etching, jewelry and enamelling at the Central School of Art and Design, before opening her own workshop in 1956. Her gold and silver jewels are all one-off pieces and are characterized by a special technique of fusing and texturing the metals rather than soldering them. Flöckinger highlights the flowing forms of the metals with semi-precious and precious stones or pearls.

Georges Fouquet (1862–1957)

In 1895 Georges Fouquet took over the jewelry business started in 1860 by his father Alphonse Fouquet (b. 1828). His pieces were chiefly in the Art Nouveau style – stylized versions of forms that drew inspiration from flora and fauna. Among the designers whose jewelry he executed were Charles Desroziers and Alphonse Mucha, the latter responsible for designing the famous snake bracelet worn by the actress Sarah Bernhardt.

Jean Fouquet (1899–1984)

Son of the jeweller *Georges Fouquet. Jean Fouquet believed that jewelry should be large and eye-catching. In the 1920s he created powerful pieces in the rigid, geometric style popular at the time. By the 1930s he was producing more curved lines. Though the House of Fouquet closed in 1936, Fouquet continued to take on private commissions and in the 1950s brought translucent enamel back into fashion.

Michaela Frey *see* **M.Frey Wille**

Lucien Gaillard (1861–1933)

French-born Lucien Gaillard took over the Paris atelier of his father, Ernest Gaillard, in 1892. He is best known for his Art Nouveau designs and for his use of Japanese techniques. Gaillard specialized in horn jewelry, including pendants, combs and hair ornaments.

Garrard & Co. Ltd

Jewelry and silverware company founded in London in 1721 by silversmith George Wickes. Garrard was appointed Crown Jeweller in the nineteenth century and its connection to the British royal family has remained strong: it has made jewelry for Queen Elizabeth II and rings for Princess Diana, Sarah Ferguson and Sophie Rhys-Jones. In 1998 it merged with *Asprey & Co. but reclaimed its independence in 2001, at which point Jade Jagger was appointed Creative Director.

Arthur J. Gaskin (1862–1928)

Born in Birmingham, UK. Gaskin studied at Birmingham School of Art, where he later taught. He designed for William Morris's Kelmscott Press, and was an illustrator, silversmith and painter, as well as a jewelry designer. His jewels are of exemplary Arts and Crafts design, often incorporating leaves, flowers and birds, and drawing inspiration from sources as various as the Italian

Renaissance and Scandinavian folk art. Gaskin also designed for *Liberty & Co. *See also* Georgina Cave Gaskin.

Georgina Cave Gaskin (1868–1934)

Georgina Gaskin, née France, studied silversmithing at Birmingham School of Art, where she met *Arthur J. Gaskin, whom she married in 1899. She specialized in jewelry and enamelling and collaborated with her husband on many pieces of jewelry.

Green & Frederick

UK company, based in Edinburgh, started in 1998 by Edward Green (b. London, UK; 1952–), previously Managing Director of both Garrard and Mappin & Webb. Green & Frederick produces 'bridge' jewelry – quality gold or platinum jewelry using cubic zirconia as a substitute for diamonds, as well as pieces using semi-precious stones.

Andrew Grima (1921–)

Born in Rome, Italy. Grima moved to London in 1926 and studied mechanical engineering at Nottingham University. In 1946 he joined H. J. Company and took over the business in 1951. Grima's early designs were traditional but in the 1960s he began to produce innovative dramatic pieces, often emphasizing unusual gemstones and incorporating objets trouvés. He was at the forefront of the decade's fashion for rough-textured gold and asymmetrical splintered forms. In 1970 he received a royal warrant and in the same year designed and made the watch collection 'About Time' for Omega. In 1986 he moved to Switzerland, where he continues to design and make jewelry with his wife JoJo and daughter Francesca.

Angela Hale (1961–)

After taking a degree in photography and film studies at Derby University, Angela Hale served as PA to Issey Miyake. She opened a costume jewelry boutique in London in 1996. Hale's jewelry is inspired by the Victorian and Art Deco periods and is handcrafted from bronze set with *Swarovski crystals. Her pieces include tiaras, hairslides/ barrettes, earrings, chokers, brooches and rings.

Miriam Haskell (1899–1981)

Born in the USA. Haskell sold jewelry from a shop in the McAlpin Hotel, New York, from 1924 until the early 1930s, when she founded her own workshop on Fifth Avenue. Favouring naturalistic themes, she designed feminine, timeless costume jewelry, frequently using 'antique' gilded surfaces, pearls and intricate beadwork. She retired and sold her company in the 1950s, but the present company still produces costume jewelry in the Haskell style.

Adolf Hildenbrand (dates unknown)

Designer working between 1900 and 1919 for *Theodor Fahrner.

Hobé Cie Ltd

William Hobé came from a family of Parisian jewellers who produced expensive, high-quality jewels. His first costume jewelry designs were created in the mid-1920s at the request of Florence

Ziegfeld for showgirls of the Ziegfeld Follies. Their success encouraged him to found the costume jewellers Hobé in New York in the 1930s. The firm was particularly known for floral brooches designed as bouquets of flowers and leaves made either in silver- or gold-plated metal, or decorated with semi-precious or glass stones.

Georg Jensen (1866–1935)
Born in Denmark. Georg Jensen studied at the School of Fine Arts of Copenhagen. Around 1901 he started to work with the artist *Mogens Ballin, making jewelry in silver and semi-precious stones. Three years later he opened a workshop in Copenhagen selling jewelry of his own design and manufacture. His pieces incorporated stylized flowers, leaves, birds and animals, somewhat in the style of Art Nouveau but with an austerity that foreshadowed the avant-garde lines of early Art Deco. After Jensen's death the firm was continued by his son Soren Georg Jensen and it became a major influence on jewelry design after the Second World War, when it employed many talented jewelry designers, including Henning Koppel and Nanna Ditzel.

Jewels by Bogoff
Jewelry house founded in Chicago in 1940 by husband-and-wife team Henry Bogoff (b. Poland; 1908–58) and Yvette Glazerman (b. Russia; dates unknown) which in the 1940s and 1950s produced high-quality imitation jewelry plated with heavy rhodium or gold and hand-set with rhinestones.

Johnny Loves Rosie
Jewelry and accessories company started in London in 1992 by Maryrose D. Monroe. Known in the mid-1990s for hair accessories such as pins, bobby pins, pony ties and flowers, it added jewelry in 1998.

Barry Kieselstein-Cord (1948–)
Born in New York, USA. Kieselstein-Cord studied at Parsons School of Design, New York University and the American Craft Institute. He founded his company, producing precious and costume jewelry and accessories, in 1972. He looks beyond fashion for inspiration and considers his work to be 'bodywork' or 'sculpture' rather than conventional jewelry. His powerful pieces, often in gold, are bold and chunky, sometimes incorporating his signature alligator design or coiled serpents.

Arthur King (1921–86)
Born in New York, USA. Arthur King discovered the technique of jewelry-making when he worked with metal as a steward in the US Merchant Navy. He opened a boutique in New York, producing one-off pieces: colourful, unconventional jewelry, using exotic materials, including fossilized prehistoric shark's tooth, Brazilian tourmalines and Biwa pearls from Japan.

Archibald Knox (1864–1933)
Born on the Isle of Man, UK. Knox made a special study of Celtic art at Douglas School of Art, Isle of Man. In 1899 he designed the first series of 'Cymric' silverware for *Liberty & Co. and soon became the firm's chief designer and the person mainly responsible for Liberty's Celtic revival. Cymric jewels were made in both silver and gold, usually set with turquoise or mother-of-pearl, or decorated with enamel, and hung with small blister pearls. Knox's designs feature the 'floating' blue and green peacock enamel – often shown behind an interlacing of silver and gold – that has almost come to symbolize English Art Nouveau jewelry. Silver jewels were often given a hand-hammered appearance.

Kutchinsky
UK jewelry company founded in the East End of London in 1893 by Polish immigrants as a watch and repair shop. Joseph Kutchinsky joined the firm in 1928 at the age of 14 and by 1958 the company was well established and had moved to the West End. New techniques developed by Kutchinsky after the Second World War included the production of a gold, silver and platinum alloy for the manufacture of jewelry. In the 1960s Kutchinsky was the first UK company to work with stones such as onyx, lapis, coral and hardstone and it created large pieces in innovative, modern designs. At the same time, and into the 1970s, it also designed large enamel pieces. In 1989 the company made the biggest jewelled egg ever produced – the pink diamond Argyle Library Egg, in the style of *Fabergé.

Christian Lacroix (1951–)
Born in Arles, France. Lacroix studied art history at Montpellier University and museum studies at the Sorbonne, Paris. He opened his couture house in Paris in 1987. His most famous jewelry design is the Byzantine-inspired cross encrusted with fake and semi-precious stones which he created in the late 1980s. His recent jewelry collections, in which silver is combined with semi-precious stones such as amethyst, garnet, rose tourmaline and agate, are more abstract and restrained. These designs range from highly modern pieces to jewelry inspired by natural, organic shapes.

Ilias Lalaounis (1920–)
Born in Athens, Greece. Descended from four generations of goldsmiths and watchmakers, Lalaounis studied economics and law at Athens University before joining the family firm, Zolatas, named after his uncle and mentor, in 1940. Lalaounis's first jewelry collections, shown in 1957, were inspired by ancient Greek art. Later collections have drawn inspiration from other cultures and from many sources, including nature and technology. In 1969, on the death of his uncle, Lalaounis established his own company. He works extensively in 22-carat gold, as well as in silver, using precious or semi-precious stones sparingly, as highlights. In 1993 he founded the Ilias Lalaounis Jewelry Museum in Athens.

René Lalique (1860–1945)
Born in Aÿ, on the Marne, France. Lalique was apprenticed to Louis Aucoq, a Parisian silversmith and jeweller. After attending art schools in Paris and London, Lalique returned to Paris where he designed for Aucoq, *Vever, *Cartier and *Boucheron. In 1886

he took over the workshop of Jules d'Estape. One of the most famous glassmakers and jewellers of the twentieth century, Lalique derived his initial success from stage jewelry made for the actress Sarah Bernhardt. He exhibited widely and achieved enormous publicity at the Paris Exposition Universelle in 1900. In 1905 he opened a shop on the Place Vendôme. His jewelry combines gold with gemstones and plique-à-jour enamelling and his designs often feature the female figure, nude or draped, with flowing hair, and sometimes with butterfly or dragonfly wings. Lalique also drew inspiration from nature – peacocks, snakes, insects and other natural forms. From 1914 he concentrated almost entirely on glass-making.

Kenneth Jay Lane (1932–)

Born in Detroit, Michigan, USA. After studying at the University of Michigan and graduating from Rhode Island School of Design, Lane joined the art department of American *Vogue* in 1954. In 1956 he left to become assistant designer at Delman Shoes and from 1958 to 1963 was associate designer for Christian Dior Shoes, New York. His first jewelry designs, in 1963, in which he utilized the rhinestones he had been using for shoe decoration, were so successful that by the following year he was running his own jewelry business. Lane makes use of plastic to simulate real gems and often sets his jewelry with opulent stones in rich colours. Considered to be one of the twentieth century's finest costume jewelry designers, his clients have included Elizabeth Taylor, Barbara Bush, Hillary Rodham Clinton and Joan Collins.

Liberty & Co.

The shop Liberty & Co. was founded in London in 1875 by Arthur Lasenby Liberty (b. Chesham, Buckinghamshire; 1843–1917), who began selling a range of decorative arts objects, chiefly from Japan and the Far East. In the late 1890s he launched a range of silverware and jewelry known as 'Cymric', in a Celtic Revival style inspired by the designs of ☆Archibald Knox. Knox was Liberty's chief designer but the firm employed many other talented artists – key figures in the Arts and Crafts and Art Nouveau movements, including Oliver Baker, Jesse M. King, David Veasey and Rex Silver – though Liberty policy was that their work was never attributed.

Maison Gripoix

Maison Gripoix, founded in the nineteenth century in Paris, specialized in the creation of high-quality handmade imitations of precious jewels. It is associated with the production of jewelry for many fashion houses, including Worth, Poiret, Piguet, Dior and Fath, but is best known for its collaboration with ☆Chanel. Susanne Gripoix (b. 1895) worked with Chanel from the mid-1920s until 1969.

Maison Vever

Parisian jewelry company founded in 1821 by Paul Vever. Paul's grandsons, Paul (1851–1915) and Henri (1854–1942) took over the business in 1874. Henri was a leading exponent of the Art Nouveau style and produced striking botanical designs. His Art Nouveau jewelry is considered second only to Lalique's. The firm employed many of the period's finest craftsmen, including Eugène Grasset (1841–1917), the Swiss painter and illustrator, who designed some of Maison Vever's most distinctive pieces.

Mappin & Webb

UK silversmiths and jewellers founded in Sheffield in 1774 by Jonathan Mappin. The first London store opened in 1849. In 1858 John Newton Mappin was joined in the business by his brother-in-law George Webb. Chiefly a silversmiths, Mappin & Webb also produces high-quality watches and jewelry. Mappin & Webb jewelry is handcrafted, using both precious and semi-precious gems. The company offers a 'Grow Your Own Diamond' service, whereby a customer can return a diamond, receive its full original purchase price, and upgrade it for a diamond of greater value.

Marina B

Jewelry company established in Geneva in 1979 by Marina Bulgari (b. Rome, Italy; 1930–). Bulgari is the daughter of the famous jeweller Constantino ☆Bulgari. She worked in the family business from an early age before setting up on her own. Among her signature pieces are perfectly fitting chokers and reversible earrings. Her jewelry often combines precious and semi-precious stones.

Marvella

Costume jewelry company founded in New York in 1906 by Sol E. Weinreich. Marvella jewelry often featured simulated pearls and faceted beads. The firm was bought by ☆Trifari in 1982 and is owned today by the ☆Monet Group Inc.

Mauboussin

French jewelry company, founded in Paris in 1827 by M. Rocher and his cousin Jean-Baptiste Noury. Georges Mauboussin, nephew of Noury, joined the firm in 1876 and later headed the company in partnership with his cousin, Marcel Goulet Mauboussin, who joined in 1896. Mauboussin's jewelry and watches are of the highest quality and are manufactured only with precious, and often rare, materials. In 1955 the firm opened a boutique to sell more affordable pieces.

Annie McLeish (dates unknown)

Turn-of-the-century freelance designer of silver clasps and belt-buckles in the ☆Liberty style.

Patricia Meyerowitz (dates unknown)

British-born jeweller and sculptor. Meyerowitz studied at the Central School of Arts and Crafts in London, and in the mid-1960s wrote her first book on jewelry and sculpture. Her jewelry has been characterized as restrained and Constructivist: she creates pieces from a number of smaller, linked elements.

M.Frey Wille

Company manufacturing jewelry in fine enamel, founded in Vienna in 1951 by the Austrian artist Michaela Frey (b. Vienna, Austria; 1926–1980). Frey developed a technique of fusing hand-applied

24-carat gold into fine enamel. M. Frey Wille jewelry focuses on art, with designs featuring Egyptian and Greco-Roman themes and artists such as Klimt and Monet. Since Frey's death the company has been headed by Friedrich Wille (b. Vienna; 1940–), a co-worker of Frey's since 1970.

Moira of Bond Street

Jewelry company founded in 1971 by Moira Cohen (b. Glasgow, Scotland; 1940–). The company initially sold nineteenth-century jewelry and jewelry of the 1960s and 1970s but Cohen soon added jewelry of her own design, taking inspiration from the forms of butterflies, dragonflies, flowers and birds. Her jewels are based on the plique-à-jour enamelling technique and use old-style settings and old, cut stones.

Monet

New York costume jewelry manufacturer, originally founded in 1929 under the name Monocraft by brothers Michael and Jay Chernow. Monet began producing jewelry in 1937. The company developed the comfortable 'friction earclip' for earrings for non-pierced ears and the 'barrel clutch' for earrings for pierced ears. In the 1980s Monet made jewelry for Yves Saint Laurent. The company is now called the Monet Group Inc. and distributes jewelry under the names Monet, *Trifari and *Marvella.

David Morris (1936–)

Born in London, UK. David Morris studied at Clark's College, London, and spent five years as an apprentice goldsmith before starting his own company in London in 1961. His son, Jeremy Morris (b. 1961), took over as head of the firm in 1983, after an apprenticeship to a goldsmith in Paris. The company is known for innovative designs and for updating themes and details from jewelry history. Recent designs include Edwardian-inspired diamond necklaces and dress watches inspired by Cubism. David Morris has had a long association with Hollywood: the company provided the diamonds for the James Bond films *Diamonds are Forever*, *Tomorrow Never Dies* and *The World is Not Enough*.

Robert Lee Morris (1947–)

Born in Nuremberg, Germany, of US parentage. After graduating from Beloit College, Wisconsin, in the late 1960s, Morris set up a crafts commune where he began to experiment with jewelry-making. His work was discovered by the owners of the artist-jeweller gallery Sculpture to Wear and in 1974 Morris moved to New York. In 1977 he opened his own gallery, Artwear, which served as a springboard for the careers of many young jewellers. Morris works closely with fashion designers. He is best known for bold organic sculptural pieces, such as the large silver cuffs and hoop earrings he designed for Donna Karan in the 1980s. He has also collaborated with Karl Lagerfeld, Michael Kors and Yohji Yamamoto, among others.

Murrle, Bennett & Co.

Founded in London in 1884 by Ernst Mürrle (b. Pforzheim,

Germany; dates unknown) and a Mr Bennett, of whom no records remain. Mürrle was interned during the First World War and, in 1916, after his repatriation to Germany, the firm was confiscated and renamed White, Redgrove and Whyte. Murrle, Bennett & Co. was a jewelry manufacturers and produced many pieces for *Liberty & Co, including some by *Archibald Knox. The company had a workshop in Pforzheim – a major jewelry-making centre – where Mürrle spent time every year working with designers *Theodor Fahrner and Wilhelm Fühner. The pieces with which the firm is most identified were taken from contemporary German designs. Characteristically restrained and geometric interpretations of Art Nouveau, they were described by the company as being 'by artists of the Modern School'.

The Napier Co.

First established in 1875 in Massachusetts, USA, as a firm selling personal objects and gifts, the firm moved to Meriden, Connecticut, in 1891 and took the name Napier in 1922 after its then-president, James H. Napier. In the 1920s The Napier Co. made its name selling copies of Paris couture jewels by Lelong, Premet, Patou, *Schiaparelli and others. Today one of America's largest costume jewellers, it has continued to respond successfully to changing fashions.

Elsa Peretti (1940–)

Born in Florence, Italy. Peretti studied interior design in Rome and worked as a fashion model before turning in 1969 to jewelry design. Sant'Angelo used some of her pieces in his shows and at the same time she began to collaborate with Halston. In 1974 she joined *Tiffany & Co. Peretti works in a variety of materials but is best known for her simple, minimalist designs in sterling silver. She also introduced the affordable and revolutionary 'Diamonds by the Yard' – thin chains interspersed with tiny diamonds.

Alfred Philippe *see* Trifari

Paloma Picasso (1949–)

Born in Paris, France. Educated at the Université de Paris at Nanterre. Picasso began as a theatrical costumier and stylist but after success with necklaces created from Folies Bergère bikinis set with rhinestones, she decided to train in jewelry design. In 1969 Yves Saint Laurent showed her jewelry with his collections. In 1980 she designed her own debut collection exclusively for *Tiffany & Co. She often works in highly polished gold and silver, combined with exotic gemstones.

Piel Frères

Parisian high-fashion jewelry firm headed at the turn of the century by Alexandre Piel, with sculptor Gabriel Stalin as artistic director. Piel Frères was known in the early twentieth century for inexpensive, high-quality, sculptural pieces, especially belt-buckles, with deeply coloured enamelling, based on Art Nouveau themes. Around 1900 the firm made jewelry in the Egyptian Revival style and created designs depicting characters from contemporary plays and opera.

In Piel Frères pieces celluloid was used in place of ivory, and copper and silver in place of gold. Around 1915–20 the firm began to create fashion jewels for Jean Patou. At the 1925 Exposition des Arts Décoratifs et Industriels Modernes, Alexandre Piel's brother, Paul, received attention for his Cubist-inspired pieces in enamelled metal fretwork.

Otto Prutscher (1880–1949)

An Austrian architect and designer, Prutscher studied from 1897 at the Kunstgewerbeschule in Vienna, where he came under the influence of Josef Hoffmann (1870–1956), founder with Kolo Moser of the Wiener Werkstätte (founded 1903; dissolved 1932). Prutscher worked as a jewelry designer for the Wiener Werkstätte, and also designed furniture, ceramics, textiles and leather goods.

Wendy Ramshaw (1939–)

Born in Sunderland, UK. Trained in industrial design at Newcastle upon Tyne College of Art and Industrial Design and at Central School of Art and Design in London. Ramshaw has been making jewelry since the 1960s out of both precious and humble materials, and has also mixed the two, as in pieces that combine paper with gold. Her pieces are interchangeable: she is especially famous for her sets of five rings, which can be worn singly or together in different combinations to vary the patterns.

Elsa Schiaparelli (1890–1973)

Born in Rome, Italy. After a period in Boston and New York, Schiaparelli moved to Paris in 1922 and opened her shop, Pour Le Sport, in 1927. She showed her first fashion collection in 1929. An original and witty couturier, Schiaparelli commissioned designs for buttons and jewelry from a range of artists, including Jean Clément, Alberto Giacometti, Salvador Dalí and Jean Cocteau. Her jewelry displays influences from many of the art movements of her day, but especially from Surrealism. In the mid-1930s she began to employ the talents of *Jean Schlumberger. It was a collaboration that would raise costume jewelry to new heights and increase its popularity and acceptability. Among Schlumberger's many innovative and amusing designs for Schiaparelli were the jewels he created to accompany her famous 'Circus' collection of 1938: clowns, acrobats, and circus horses' heads made of gilt metal or Venetian glass. Schiaparelli closed her house in 1954.

Jean Schlumberger (1907–1987)

Born in Mulhouse, Alsace, France. After initial study for a career in banking, Schlumberger went to Paris in the 1920s and began making pieces of costume jewelry from glass beads and porcelain flowers found in flea-markets. These caught the attention of the fashion designer *Elsa Schiaparelli, who commissioned him to make buttons and costume jewelry. Schlumberger emigrated in the early 1940s to New York, where he opened his own business in partnership with Nicholas Bongard, nephew of the designer Paul Poiret. Schlumberger's designs of flowers, starfish, birds, angels and other motifs (the sea-horse was his signature design) brought him success throughout the 1940s and 1950s. In 1956 he joined *Tiffany & Co. as designer and vice-president. His designs of the late 1950s, 1960s and 1970s are rich and fantastic, incorporating his favourite organic subject matter and with a daring use of colour and an inventive mix of precious and semi-precious stones, gold and enamels.

Swarovski

Austrian company founded in 1895 in Wattens, in the Tyrol, by Daniel Swarovski (b. Georgenthal, Austria; 1862–1956). In 1892 Swarovski patented a machine for cutting glass gemstones with perfect precision. The company makes high-quality rhinestones, cut crystals and other glass-related items. It began a line of rhinestone costume jewelry in 1977.

Raymond Templier (1891–1968)

Templier came from a family of Parisian jewellers (the firm Maison Templier had been started by his grandfather Charles Templier in 1849). His designs are in the Art Deco style, strongly geometric but featuring precious stones in some abundance. He achieved success with pieces in platinum or silver combined with onyx and other dark stones – a typically black-and-white Art Deco combination.

Tiffany & Co.

Founded in New York in 1837 by Charles Lewis Tiffany (1812–1902) and John B. Young as a stationers and fancy goods store. In 1841 it expanded into jewelry, buying in pieces from Paris, and by 1848 was manufacturing its own jewelry. In 1868 the firm merged with the silversmiths Edward C. Moore & Co., and Moore – a designer for Tiffany since 1851 – was instrumental in introducing Japanese styles. With the death of Charles Lewis Tiffany, his son, Louis Comfort Tiffany (1848–1933), joined the company. The latter's talents extended to many aspects of the decorative arts, including jewelry, glass-making and silverware. The firm produced greatly admired Art Nouveau jewelry designs and successfully followed the changing styles of the 1930s and 1940s. In 1955 Tiffany's was bought by Walter Hoving and the following year Hoving invited the jeweller *Jean Schlumberger to join Tiffany's as chief designer. Tiffany's success has been built not only on its own design expertise but also on its ability to recognize talent. Other designers who have worked under the Tiffany umbrella include Donald Claflin, *Angela Cummings, *Elsa Peretti and *Paloma Picasso.

Alexander Tillander (1837–1918)

After an early apprenticeship with two goldsmiths in Tsarskoe Selo and St Petersburg, Helsinki-born Alexander Tillander started producing simple gold bangles. He gradually built up his workshop, adding rings, brooches with matching earrings, cufflinks and studs to his output and acquiring a reputation for high-quality workmanship. In the early twentieth century the firm began to enjoy the patronage of various branches of European royalty. Alexander Jnr (b. 1907) later joined his father. After the Revolution the House of Tillander was re-established in Helsinki. Oskar Pihl was chief designer until his death in 1957. The firm continues today.

Jeanne Toussaint *see* **Cartier**

Trifari

American jewelry manufacturing company founded in 1910 by Gustavo Trifari. Leo Krussman joined Trifari in 1917 and Carl Fishel in 1918, at which point the company was renamed Trifari, Krussman & Fishel. The three men became known as 'The Diamanté Kings', producing highly successful imitations of the most popular precious jewelry of the time. Initially offering Art Deco designs, they followed changing fashions over the decades, bringing out cocktail jewelry in the 1930s, a legendary series of 'jelly-belly' animals in the 1940s, and shiny diamanté-studded pieces (often parures) in the 1950s. Alfred Philippe, the highly original designer who had created pieces for *Cartier and *Van Cleef & Arpels, was employed by Trifari from 1930 to the 1950s. Mamie Eisenhower commissioned Trifari to design faux pearl and diamanté parures for the presidential inaugurations of 1952 (designed by Alfred Philippe) and 1956. Trifari is now owned by the *Monet Group Inc.

Van Cleef & Arpels

French jewelry firm founded in Paris in 1906 by Julien Arpels (1884–1964), Charles Arpels (1880–1951) and their brother-in-law Alfred van Cleef (1873–1938). They were joined by Louis Arpels (1886–1976) in 1912. In the 1930s the firm designed a new type of vanity case known as a minaudière, and developed invisible settings that could be used to create mosaic-like surfaces of precious stones. In 1954 the firm opened a boutique department offering less expensive jewels.

Line Vautrin (*c.* 1918–97)

Born in France. At the age of 20 Line Vautrin began making jewelry which she sold house-to-house. In 1937 she opened a shop in Paris, offering jewelry, belts, shoes, buttons, etc. Her first bestseller was a gilt-bronze pendant showing Adam and Eve in the Garden of Eden. An artist-jeweller of great wit and imagination, Vautrin created bold, primitive designs on a variety of themes, including nature – birds, leaves, flowers, fish, etc. – and the lives of the saints. She worked almost exclusively in gilt bronze.

Fulco di Verdura (1898–1978)

Born in Palermo, Sicily. In 1927 Verdura started working in Paris for *Chanel as a textile designer but soon turned to jewelry design. He created two of Chanel's signature pieces – a pair of pearl earrings surrounded by gold rope and two wide enamelled cuff bracelets encrusted with jewelled Maltese crosses. In 1934 he moved to New York and after a period designing for the jeweller Paul Flato he opened his own shop in 1939. Verdura's work exerted a considerable influence on later jewellers. He was the first to prefer coloured gemstones and gold to platinum and diamonds and also the first to incorporate real pebbles and shells in his designs. He favoured bright, colourful enamels, used both precious and semi-precious stones in the same setting and frequently took inspiration from nature: motifs common in his pieces include shells, feathers, wings and leaves. His twisted baroque pearls and gold chains were particularly popular.

Vever *see* **Maison Vever**

Wartski

Wartski was established in 1865 in Bangor, North Wales, by Morris Wartski. The firm moved to Llandudno in 1907 and, after the marriage of Wartski's daughter to Emanuel Snowman (1887–1970), relocated to London in 1911. Until the 1920s Wartski specialized in gem-set jewelry and antique silver but after a visit to Russia by Snowman in 1925 it began to stock items of Russian origin, including *Fabergé eggs. Snowman's son, Kenneth Snowman, became chairman of the firm on his father's death. The firm's directors – Kenneth Snowman, Geoffrey Munn and Katherine Purcell – have published a number of scholarly works on jewelry. Wartski has a number of royal warrants and is known for its exceptional collection of antique jewelry.

Harry Winston (1896–1978)

Born in New York, USA. Winston, the son of a watch-jeweller, began his jewelry-making career in Los Angeles at the age of 15. He established Harry Winston, Inc. in 1932. A wholesaler, dealer and cutter of diamonds, Winston specialized in important stones, usually in simple settings. Known as the 'King of Diamonds', he handled or owned a large proportion of the world's most famous stones, including the Hope diamond. On his death the firm was taken over by his son, Ronald Winston (b. 1941).

Philippe Wolfers (1858–1929)

Born in Brussels, Belgium. Grandson of the founder of Wolfers Frères, Belgium's leading jewelry company (established 1850), Philippe Wolfers joined the family business in 1890, along with his brothers Max (1859–1953) and Robert (1867–1959), but started his own workshop in the same year. He is remembered for an outstanding series of Art Nouveau pieces. He stopped making jewelry in 1910.

Sources for 20th Century Jewelry

Baker, Lillian, *Art Nouveau and Art Deco Jewelry: An Identification and Value Guide*, Paducah, Kentucky, 1981

—, *Fifty Years of Collectible Fashion Jewelry 1925–1975*, Paducah, Kentucky, 1986

Ball, Joanne Dubbs, *Costume Jewelers: The Golden Age of Design*, West Chester, Penn., 1990

—, *Jewelry of the Stars: Creations from Joseff of Hollywood*, West Chester, Penn., 1991

Battle, Dee, and Alayne Lesser, *The Best of Bakelite and Other Plastic Jewelry*, Atglen, Penn., 1996

Becker, Vivienne, *Antique and 20th Century Jewellery*, London, 1987

—, *Fabulous Fakes: The History of Fantasy and Fashion Jewellery*, London, 1988

—, *The Jewellery of René Lalique*, London, 1987

—, *Rough Diamonds: The Butler & Wilson Collection*, London, 1990

Bell, Jeanenne, *Answers to Questions about Old Jewelry: 1840–1950*, Iola, Wisc., 1999

Black, J. Anderson, *A History of Jewels*, London, 1974

Brunialti, Carla Ginelli, and Roberto Brunialti, *American Costume Jewelry: 1935–1950*, Milan, 1997

Burkholz, Matthew L., and Linda Lichtenberg Kaplan, *Copper Art Jewelry: A Different Lustre*, West Chester, Penn., 1992

Clements, Monica Lynn, and Patricia Rosser Clements, *Avon: Collectible Fashion Jewelry and Awards*, Atglen, Penn., 1998

—, *Sarah Coventry Jewelry*, Atglen, Penn., 1999

Cumo, Carlo, and Claude Mazloum, *Jewelry Gem by Gem: Masters and Materials*, Rome, 1996

Ditmer, Judy, *Turning Wooden Jewelry*, Atglen, Penn., 1994

Dormer, Peter, and Ralph Turner, *The New Jewelry: Trends and Traditions*, London, 1986

Drutt, Helen W., and Peter Dormer, *Jewelry of Our Time*, London, 1995

Dufrene, Maurice, *305 Authentic Art Nouveau Jewelry Designs*, London, 1985

Edwards, Juliette, *Powder Compacts: A Collector's Guide*, London, 2000

Ettinger, Roseann, *Forties and Fifties Popular Jewelry*, Atglen, Penn., 1994

—, *Popular Jewelry 1840–1940*, West Chester, Penn., 1990

—, *Popular Jewelry of the '60s, '70s and '80s*, Atglen, Penn., 1997

Farneti Cera, Deanna, *Costume Jewellery*, Milan, 1997

—, *The Jewels of Miriam Haskell*, Woodbridge, Suffolk, and Milan, 1997

Gere, Charlotte, and Geoffrey C. Munn, *Jewellery: Pre-Raphaelite to Arts and Crafts*, London, 1999

Gilhooley, Derren, and Simon Costin (eds. Alexandra Bradley and Gavin Fernandes), *Unclasped: Contemporary British Jewellery*, London, 1997

Grasso, Tony, *Bakelite Jewelry: A Collector's Guide*, New Jersey, 1996

Hinks, Peter, *Twentieth Century British Jewellery: 1900–1980*, London, 1983

Hughes, Graham, *A Pictorial History of Gems and Jewellery*, London, 1978

Hurel, Roselyne, and Diana Scarisbrick, *Chaumet, Paris: Two Centuries of Fine Jewellery*, Paris, 1998

James, Duncan, *Old Jewellery*, Princes Risborough, 1989

Jargstorf, Sibylle, *Baubles, Buttons, and Beads: The Heritage of Bohemia*, Atglen, Penn., 1993

—, *Glass in Jewelry: Hidden Artistry in Glass*, West Chester, Penn., 1991

Kelley, Lyngerda, and Nancy Schiffer, *Costume Jewelry: The Great Pretenders*, West Chester, Penn., 1987

Lane, Kenneth Jay, and Harrice Simons Miller, *Faking It*, New York, 1996

Loring, John, *Tiffany's 20th Century*, New York, 1997

Mascetti, Daniela, and Amanda Triossi, *Earrings from Antiquity to the Present*, London, 1990

Mauriès, Patrick, *Jewelry by Chanel*, London, 1993

Mazloum, Claude, *Jewellery and Gemstones*, Rome, 1998

McCreight, Tim, *Jewellery: Fundamentals of Metalsmithing*, London, 1998

Mueller, Laura M., *Collector's Encyclopedia of Compacts, Carryalls and Face Powder Boxes*, Paducah, Kentucky, 1994

Mulvagh, Jane, *Costume Jewelry in Vogue*, London, 1988

Nadelhoffer, Hans, *Cartier: Jewelers Extraordinary*, London, 1984

Néret, Gilles, *Boucheron: Four Generations of A World-Renowned Jeweler*, New York, 1988

Newman, Harold, *An Illustrated Dictionary of Jewelry*, London, 1981

Phillips, Clare, *Jewelry: From Antiquity to the Present*, London, 1996

—, *Jewels and Jewellery*, London, 2000

Pullee, Caroline, *20th Century Jewellery*, London, 1990

Raulet, Sylvie, *Art Deco Jewelry*, London, 1984

Sataloff, Joseph, and Alison Richards, *The Pleasure of Jewelry and Gemstones*, London, 1975

Scarisbrick, Diana, *Jewellery*, London, 1998

—, *Jewellery Source Book*, London, 1998

Schiffer, Nancy, *Fun Jewelry*, Atglen, Penn., 1997

Shields, Jody, *All That Glitters: The Glory of Costume Jewelry*, New York, 1987

Snowman, A. Kenneth (ed.), *The Master Jewelers*, London, 1990

Taylor, Gerald, *Finger Rings: From Ancient Egypt to the Present Day*, London, 1978

Tolkien, Tracy, and Henrietta Wilkinson, *A Collector's Guide to Costume Jewelry: Key Styles and How to Recognise Them*, London, 1997

Von Hase-Schmundt, Ulrike, and Christianne Weber and Ingeborg Becker, *Theodor Fahrner Jewelry: Between Avant-Garde and Tradition*, West Chester, Penn., 1991

Ward, Anne, and John Cherry, Charlotte Gere and Barbara Cartlidge, *The Ring: From Antiquity to the Twentieth Century*, London, 1981

West, Janice, *Made to Wear: Creativity in Contemporary Jewellery*, London, 1998

Willcox, Donald J., *New Design in Jewelry*, New York, 1970